LONG TERM REHABILITATION FOR STROKE AND TBI

BUILDING A COMMUNITY

LONG TERM REHABILITATION FOR STROKE AND TBI

BUILDING A COMMUNITY

Beverly Greer

Chief Executive Officer
Stroke Recovery Center

Copyright © 2011 by Beverly Greer.

Library of Congress Control Number: 2011917362
ISBN: Hardcover   978-1-4653-7126-3
               Softcover   978-1-4653-7125-6
               E-book   978-1-4653-7127-0

All rights reserved. No part of this book may be reproduced or transmitted in any form or by any means, electronic or mechanical, including photocopying, recording, or by any information storage and retrieval system, without permission in writing from the copyright owner.

This book was printed in the United States of America.

To order additional copies of this book, contact:
Xlibris Corporation
1-888-795-4274
www.Xlibris.com
Orders@Xlibris.com

The book is dedicated to Carol Sue Rosenthal Konoski, the least-handicapped handicapped person I have ever met, for teaching me to look beyond the disability.

Treat people as if they were what they ought to be, and help them become what they are capable of being.

—Goethe

CONTENTS

Introduction ix

Section I: Stroke and/or TBI 1

Chapter I: What You Need to Know About Strokes and TBI 3
    What Happens When One Has a Stroke or TBI 6
    How Do People React to Having a Stroke? 9
    Possible Stroke Problems 10
    Possible Traumatic Brain Injury Problems 13
    Acute Rehabilitation—Who Does What? 16
    One Other Issue 23

Chapter II: Where Do You Get Help? 26
    Families and Friends 27
    Community and Organizations 29

Chapter III: Caregivers and Loved Ones 32
    Caregivers and Patients 33
    Caregiving Problems of Families and Loved Ones 35

Chapter IV: Stroke Recovery Center Options 39
    Let's Talk Research 39
    Success Factors 44

Chapter V: Alternative Therapies 49

Section II: The Stroke Recovery Center 51

Chapter I: History 53

Chapter II: Philosophy 55

Chapter III: Programs and Services Provided 58
    Exercise Therapy 58
    Speech and Language Therapy 61

    Recreational Therapy 62
    The Food Program 68

Chapter IV: What Is Needed for a Stroke Recovery Center? 70
    Patients 70
    Physical Needs 71
    Staffing 71
    Constraints 72
    Development: Raising Money 73
    The Importance of Leadership: Building a Board 75

Chapter V: Barriers to Development 77
    Catch 22 for CBOs 77
    Government and/or Public Financing 78

Section III: Advocacy 81
    Economics of Stroke Recovery 83
    Community Advocacy 85
    Advocating for a Stroke Recovery Center 85
    Models of Care 88
    Social Networking and Advocacy 91

Afterword 93

Notes 95

References 97

Sample Menu 167

Sample Activities Calendar 168

Website 170

Stats Report 171

Bibliography 173

Index 175

INTRODUCTION

Stroke survivors and other brain-injured survivors (including those with traumatic brain injuries, aneurisms, and the like) share the catastrophic lack of insurance coverage for long-term rehabilitation. The standard emanating from Medicare allows for some physical therapy and, if needed, speech therapy to be paid for; however, the visits are doomed to end in what may be as little as thirty days—perhaps extending to ninety days. At this point, further recovery is left to the survivor's will and his pocketbook. What this means is that those people who lack the resources to hire professionals fall through the cracks and languish at home or in institutions with little to no hope of further improvement in their quality of life. They may be a significant burden to their families, they may cause a lack of productivity in the household that can result in financial catastrophe, or they may become a financial burden to society as a whole.

What this book is designed to do is to detail the issues that stroke and TBI survivors and their families face as the safety net collapses around them. Additionally, we will introduce the option for continued treatment that has proven effective both in quality and cost—evidence-based practice at the Stroke Recovery Center. In presenting the best practice methodology and financing options and opportunities, we are hoping to encourage providers to see the advantages to providing comparable services to this underserved population.

The Stroke Recovery Center has been helping people recover from the effects of stroke and TBI for the last thirty-two years—all services are free. While originally started by a physician, the programs have evolved into a mixture of clinical and nonclinical services that include physical, speech, and recreational therapies. We see over three hundred people each year, many of whom stay with us for years as they continue to recover from the deficits that they have suffered. We see the patients, we see the families, and we see the ongoing frustrations, the issues, and the problems that have to be faced and that have to be dealt with to keep moving forward to a full recovery. We understand the depression, anxiety, bipolar illness, and anger that can accompany the brain injury. We understand the helplessness and we understand the hopelessness that can happen with brain damage. However, on the other hand, we see the celebration, the hope, and the joy—those small miracles—that come from improvements however small and the regaining of some control over activities of daily living.

In the first section of the book, we will look to others for their experiences to detail the issues that the patients and their families face. Using both the experiences of patients at the Stroke Recovery Center and experiences of those who have chosen to write about their own struggles, we can better understand the unmet needs and the ineffectiveness of current practices. It is important to understand that stroke is a life-altering event for both the survivor and their family. The issues that the caregivers face have as much weight in the problem and solution as a whole as do the survivors. It is also important to look at the current level of resources open to survivors and their families despite their severe limitations.

In the second section of the book, we will talk about the Stroke Recovery Center and how one starts a center like ours. This section will detail how the issues that are discussed in section 1 of the book are dealt with to build the community that is necessary to give hope and support for continued recovery. All the information you need (including the philosophy, the treatment plans, the scheduling, the motivating, the food, the fund-raising, and the building of a board of directors) is included to deal with the survivors and the families that support you. Since all services are provided for free, we recognize sustainability is the major issue in the provision of services on a widespread basis. Fund-raising for operations is a difficult and specialized endeavor, one that requires full-time staff and diligent attention. As health-care reform proceeds, it appears there are some alternative sources of revenue that will allow for stroke recovery centers to take their places as safety net providers for chronic care.

In the last segment of the book, we will discuss health-care reform. We build the case for more centers of help and hope. We show how the cost curve for chronic care and the quality curve are both affected. As health-care costs continue to soar, all of us need to understand the high cost of chronic care (both physically and emotionally) and, once alternate care scenarios are proven, advocate for and insist upon help and hope for those citizens of our country who need that additional help. Recognizing that free services are very difficult to sustain, this section will also point out opportunities for stroke centers to fit into the continuum of care that currently exists for a number of differing organizations and present the argument for funding that is needed to expand the current service offering to stroke and TBI survivors throughout the country. There are models of care that are being incorporated into health-care reform that present an opportunity to fund and sustain long-term care to this underserved population.

I want to give a special thanks to all the patients and families who have participated at the Stroke Recovery Center over the years and allowed us to share their stories. Additionally, I am very grateful to my associate and friend, Lois H. Kahn-Feurer, PhD, who not only gives off herself as a volunteer at the Stroke Recovery Center but also assists me in understanding the special needs of the brain-injured patients and their families.

Margaret Meade said, "Never doubt that a small group of thoughtful, committed people can change the world. Indeed, it is the only thing that ever has." Armed with this information, we have the opportunity to change the world for this underserved and forgotten group of fellow citizens.

SECTION I

STROKE AND/OR TBI

CHAPTER I

WHAT YOU NEED TO KNOW ABOUT STROKES AND TBI

Stroke is the leading cause of adult disability in the United States. Every year, about 800,000 people have a stroke. Of those, almost 600,000 are first-time incidents with the remaining being recurring episodes. Stroke is the fourth leading cause of death in the United States. Strokes leave some 65% of survivors with one or more deficits that are severe enough to interfere with activities of daily living, but not severe enough to require institutionalization. What this means is that every year, over 500,000 people join the pool of stroke survivors in need of long-term care. Survival rates vary from 1.8 to 7.4 years. It is estimated that there are in excess of 3 million people living with the ravages of stroke. As the population ages, this problem will only become greater; and with the safety net shrinking even further each year, long-term chronic-care costs threaten to overwhelm the health-care system as a whole.

Statistically, more women have strokes each year than men. Because women live longer than men and the incidence of stroke increases with age, more women die each year from stroke—60% of deaths are women. Survival times from the time of the first stroke vary from a high of 7.4 years for women ages 60–69 to a low of 1.8 years for men ages 80+.

There are basically two different types of strokes: hemorrhagic and ischemic. Hemorrhagic strokes may be either intracerebral or subarachnoid. The ischemic stroke accounts for 87% of all strokes. This is a blockage to the brain caused by a blood clot. The area blocked from normal blood flow begins to die, and the damage that ensues result in the deficits that we see in survivors. These deficits occur in the area of the blood restriction and, therefore, may result in singular or multiple problems. The result of the intracerebral hemorrhage is much the same, except the damage is caused by a blood vessel breaking or seeping with a resultant decrease of blood to a specific portion of the brain. Only 10% of strokes are of this kind. Subarachnoid hemorrhages are far rarer—only 3%—and 50% are fatal. This type of stroke involves bleeding between the brain and the tissues that cover the brain. Finally, we cannot forget the TIA or transient ischemic attack, referred to as a ministroke, which lasts less than twenty-four hours. About 15% of strokes are preceded by a TIA, and people who have had a TIA have a 10-year stroke risk of 18%.

TBI or traumatic brain injury is also a leading cause of death and disability. It differs from a stroke in that it is usually the result of a trauma of some sort. Fatalities in the United States from TBI are caused by vehicle accidents—34%, firearms—39%, falls—10%, and others—17%. Every year, about 2 million people suffer a TBI. About 500,000 are hospitalized. The greatest number of TBIs occur in people aged 15–24. TBI is more common in men.

Statistics are dry numbers that do nothing to tell the story behind the devastation that can come from a stroke or a TBI. What they can tell us is that if we have not had a stroke or a TBI ourselves, it is likely that we will know someone who has. And, as we age, that likelihood will increase, especially for stroke. So if the possibility increases that we might have a stroke or that someone we love might have a stroke and require care, we should look at the experience of having a stroke and what happens after the incident: what are the most significant problems early on, what are the most significant problems later, and where to get help.

Having worked for a number of years with stroke and TBI survivors at the Stroke Recovery Center, from a nonclinical point of view, we can say if you have seen one stroke, you have seen one stroke. This is because the damage to the brain varies according to the area affected as well as what we believe are the various ways individuals process information. Of course, there are common diagnoses for aphasia, hemiparalysis, vision problems, mental health problems, and the like that may occur with the incident, but we also see a wide variation in how the damage is expressed and how individuals react to it.

If a stroke is treated early—in the first few hours after the incident—it is possible to minimize the damage. The trick is to recognize that a stroke is occurring. The signs may be subtle: sudden numbness or weakness of arm, face, or leg, especially on one side of the body; sudden trouble in speaking or understanding; sudden trouble in seeing or blurring of vision; sudden trouble in walking; sudden dizziness; sudden loss of balance or coordination; or a sudden very severe headache with no known cause. Of those symptoms, the headache, which may signal an aneurism or hemorrhagic stroke, is the most dramatic and easily recognized as a call for emergency help. The other symptoms may be easily misinterpreted or excused. We have had numerous reports from our clients over the years of ignoring the symptoms or having the symptoms misinterpreted. One of our clients suffered from dizziness and weakness while picking up food for his family at a local fast-food outlet. He got to his car and was summarily stopped by the police. They took him into custody for drunk-driving and called his wife. She told them to keep him overnight if he was drunk to teach him a lesson. He did not get treatment until the following day. Another story that was widely reported on NPR told of a writer who woke up one morning to his early newspaper only to find that the paper was written in Croatian. Since he did not read Croatian, it is not really clear how he recognized that the particular Cyrillic was Croatian, but he thought that someone was playing a trick on him. He went into his library and picked up a book and found that the book was also in the same language, and he was unable to read it. As a well-educated fellow, it was at this point he realized that he had a problem and needed help; he called 911, and he was taken to the hospital.

We have a policy here at the Stroke Recovery Center that we tell to all our clients—to those who call in for information and for those community members who we educate with our outreach programs. If you have any doubt at all, call 911 or go to the ER. The best thing you can hear is that you did not have a stroke. If you have had a stroke, early treatment to dissolve the blood clot will expedite recovery and minimize damages. Err on the side of caution—the damages may be severe, and we need all the help we can get.

TBI does not have the same identification problems since it is the result of a traumatic occurrence. While most traumatic brain injuries result in widespread damage to the brain because the brain ricochets inside the skull during the impact of an accident, there may be some injuries that are not identified, such as sports injuries that may not be treated as serious but may result in long-term problems. When the brain is in trauma, diffuse axonal injuries may occur when the nerve cells are torn from one another. Localized damage may also occur when the brain bounces against the skull. The brain stem, frontal lobe, and temporal lobes are particularly vulnerable to this because of their location near bony protrusions.

WHAT HAPPENS WHEN ONE HAS A STROKE OR TBI

To understand better what actually occurs when you have a stroke, it is best to listen to the experiences of those who have had strokes and who have written about it or talked about it here at the center. There have been numerous books written about the experience of having a stroke and the problems with recovery. Most of which have been written by hemorrhagic stroke sufferers.

One of the most touching and horrifying accounts of a catastrophic stroke was written by a Frenchman, Jean-Dominique Bauby, who awoke from a coma to a locked-in syndrome. The book that he wrote about his experience, *The Diving Bell and the Butterfly*, was written entirely by his communication with his speech therapist by the blinking of one eye to indicate the letter of alphabet. Using this method, Jean was able to tell of his experience waking entrapped in his body, unable to move or communicate. His body is the diving bell he speaks of, and the butterfly is his imagination that frees him, if only momentarily, from his prison. This poignant account was made into a movie that was subsequently nominated for an Academy Award.

He wrote, "I had never even heard of the brain stem. I've since learned that it is an essential component of our internal computer, the inseparable link between the brain and the spinal cord. I was brutally introduced to this vital piece of anatomy when a cerebrovascular accident took my brain stem out of action… you survive, but you survive with what is known so aptly as 'locked-in' syndrome. Paralyzed from head to toe, the patient, his mind intact, is imprisoned inside his own body, unable to speak pr move… of course, the party chiefly concerned is the last to hear the good news. I had twenty days of deep coma and several weeks of grogginess and somnolence before I truly appreciated the extent of damage."[1]

Fortunately, most stroke survivors do not awaken to locked-in syndrome, but they do awake to a new world that is vastly different from the one they left. One of the most detailed accounts of the effects of stroke has been written by Jill Bolte Taylor, PhD. Dr. Taylor was a brain researcher at Harvard prior to her stroke and, because of her knowledge, was able to recount details that most of us as laypeople would not notice or remember as significant. In a speech to TEDS, Dr. Taylor said that when she realized she was having a stroke, she thought, *I'm a brain researcher, I'm having a stroke. How cool is that!*

In her book *My Stroke of Insight,* she states, "It really was fascinating for me to watch and experience myself during those earliest stages of recovery. Because of my academics, I intellectually conceptualized my body as a compilation of various neurological programs, but it wasn't until this experience with stroke that I really understood that we all have the ability to lose pieces of ourselves one program at a time.... Imagine, if you will, what it would feel like to have each of your natural faculties systematically peeled away from your consciousness. First, imagine you lose your ability to make sense of sound coming in through your ears. You are not deaf; you simply hear all sounds as chaos and noise. Second, remove your ability to see the defined forms of any objects in your space. You are not blind, you simply cannot see three-dimensionally, or identify color. You have not ability to track an object in motion or distinguish clear boundaries between objects. In addition, common smells become so amplified that they overwhelm you."[2]

The constant theme to be heard from everyone's recollections is that the poststroke world is not the one that existed the day prior. "I tried to ask what was wrong with me... what came out of my mouth made no sense and... my left side refused to move... I became very frightened... my left hand was like a poor little injured bird, unable to move."[3] "My left arm was completely paralyzed. Most of my left leg was paralyzed. My trunk muscles wouldn't respond. I couldn't sit up. My right arm and leg responded to my thoughts of moving them, but they were wildly uncoordinated and wandered all over the place. My swallowing reflex was gone… speech heavily slurred… eyes wouldn't focus. My ability to control my emotional expression was shot."[4] Loss of feeling in one side of the body, loss of half of the visual field, confusion, fear, anger, and inability to control one's emotions are common to stroke survivors. Loss of communication skills, loss of swallowing reflexes, loss of control over bodily functions, loss of short- or long-term memory, loss of sequential thinking skills, and on and on. Each stroke or traumatic brain injury takes its own toll, dependent upon the site and the extent of damage to the brain. The self who was the day before is no longer there. As the partners of a patient at the Stroke Recovery Center whose loved one had been very athletic (an ardent mountain climber and biker) said, "It was as if Supergirl fell out of the sky."

Traumatic brain injury (TBI) can result in many of the same symptoms as stroke. Mild Traumatic Brain Injury (MTBI) is characterized by one or more of the following symptoms: a brief loss of consciousness, loss of memory immediately before or after the injury, any alteration in mental state at the time of the accident, or focal neurological deficits. In many MTBI cases, the person seems fine on the surface yet continues to endure chronic functional problems. Some people suffer long-term effects of MTBI known as postconcussion syndrome (PCS). Persons suffering from PCS and other more severe TBI can experience significant changes in cognition or the ability to concentrate and remember; in sensory processing or the ability to understand sight, hearing, touch, taste, and smell; and communication or the ability to express and understand. Changes in personality or mental health issues such as depression, anxiety, aggression, and social inappropriateness may also occur. Others with MTBI experience a transient or short-term interruption followed by spontaneous recovery.

Moderate TBI is considered when there is a loss of consciousness that lasts for more than thirty minutes but less than twenty-four hours and memory loss after the traumatic event, called post-traumatic amnesia or PTA, lasting for twenty-four hours to seven days. Severe TBI is classified based on a loss of consciousness that lasts for more than twenty-four hours, PTA lasting for seven days or longer, and a deeper coma.

In terms of TBI, the damage may be more diffuse and involve the brain stem. The brain stem is located at the base of the brain, and aside from regulating basic arousal and regulatory functions, the brain stem is involved in attention and short-term memory. Trauma to this area can lead to disorientation, frustration, and anger. The limbic system, higher up in the brain than the brain stem, helps regulate emotions. Connected to the limbic system are the temporal lobes that are involved in many cognitive skills such as memory and language. Damage to the temporal lobes or seizures in this area have been associated with a number of behavioral disorders. The frontal lobe is almost always injured due to its large size and its location near the front of the cranium. The frontal lobe is involved in many cognitive functions and is considered our emotional and personality control center. Damage to this area can result in decreased judgment and increased impulsivity.

Attention to and rehabilitation for all levels of TBI have increased recently with the prominence of traumatic brain injury in returning veterans. Adjustment to civilian life can be complicated by the diagnosis and treatment of a TBI. The VA has implemented a single point of entry for care for these veterans. The average age of a veteran today is reported to be twenty-four, which can bring additional biological and psychological matters into their rehabilitation.

HOW DO PEOPLE REACT TO HAVING A STROKE?

"I was saddened by the inability of the medical community to know how to communicate with someone in my condition.... I wanted my doctors to focus on how my brain was working rather than whether it worked according to their criteria or timetable."[5] These words of Dr. Taylor's mirror those written by many who have had strokes and suffered the same frustration of trying to communicate in those first days following a stroke or TBI.

Jean-Dominique Bauby wrote about the hospital staff. "The hospital staff are of two kinds: the majority, who would not dream of leaving the room without first attempting to decipher my SOS messages; and the less conscientious minority, who make their getaway pretending not to notice my distress signals.... Later... as time cooled my fiercest rages, I got to know them better. They carried out as best they could their delicate mission: to ease our burden a little when our crosses bruised our shoulders too painfully."[6] "I was so mad for so long that there were many times I said 'no' to everything.

I seemed to dislike a lot of people who were trying to help me. I was just mad at the world. I was so frustrated."[7]

The frustration that is felt is well expressed by Julia Fox Garrison in her book: *Don't Leave Me This Way*. She says that the number one poststroke indignity is "listening to people speak about you as if you are not in the room."[8] "Isn't this (the hospital) a place where people come to get help recovering from whatever it is that has, you know, befallen them? If that's so, then why does everyone act like I'm an inconvenience? Or a description? Or a line on a chart?"[9]

While as a patient you are undergoing the trauma of discovering this new and frightening status of your body, your emotions, and your thoughts, simultaneously, rehabilitative therapy will begin. Often within twenty-four to forty-eight hours after the stroke, the first goals will involve promoting independent movement because many patients are paralyzed or seriously weakened. Patients are prompted to change positions frequently while lying in bed and to engage in passive or active range-of-motion exercises to strengthen their stroke-impaired limbs. (Passive range-of-motion exercises are those in which the therapist actively helps the patient move a limb repeatedly, whereas active exercises are performed by the patient with no physical assistance from the therapist.) Patients progress from sitting up and transferring between the bed and a chair to standing, bearing their own weight, and walking with or without assistance. Rehabilitation nurses and physical therapists help patients perform progressively more complex and demanding tasks, such as bathing, dressing, and using a toilet, and they encourage patients to begin using their stroke-impaired limbs while engaging in those tasks. Beginning to reacquire the ability to carry out these basic activities of daily living represents the first stage in a stroke survivor's return to functional independence.

POSSIBLE STROKE PROBLEMS

As we have talked about before, the types and degrees of disability that follow a stroke depend upon which area of the brain is damaged. Generally, stroke can cause five types of disabilities that we will detail below: paralysis or problems controlling movement, sensory disturbances including pain, problems using or understanding language, problems with thinking and memory, and emotional disturbances.

Paralysis or Problems Controlling Movement (Motor Control)

Paralysis is one of the most common disabilities resulting from stroke. The paralysis is usually on the side of the body opposite the side of the brain damaged by stroke and may affect the face, an arm, a leg, or the entire side of the body. This one-sided paralysis is called hemiplegia (one-sided weakness is called hemiparesis). Stroke patients with hemiparesis or hemiplegia may have difficulty with everyday activities such as walking or grasping objects. Some stroke patients have problems with swallowing, called dysphagia, due to damage to the part of the brain that controls the muscles for swallowing. Damage to a lower part of the brain, the cerebellum, can affect the body's ability to coordinate movement, a disability called ataxia, leading to problems with body posture, walking, and balance.

Sensory Disturbances Including Pain

Stroke patients may lose the ability to feel touch, pain, temperature, or position—their bearings. Sensory deficits may also hinder the ability to recognize objects that patients are holding and can even be severe enough to cause loss of recognition of one's own limb. Some stroke patients experience pain, numbness, or odd sensations of tingling or prickling in paralyzed or weakened limbs, a condition known as paresthesia.

Stroke survivors frequently have a variety of chronic pain syndromes resulting from stroke-induced damage to the nervous system (neuropathic pain). Patients who have a seriously weakened or paralyzed arm commonly experience moderate to severe pain that radiates outward from the shoulder. Most often, the pain results from a joint becoming immobilized due to lack of movement, and the tendons and ligaments around the joint become fixed in one position. This is commonly called a frozen joint; passive movement at the joint in a paralyzed limb is essential to prevent painful freezing and to allow easy movement if and when voluntary motor strength returns. In some stroke patients, pathways for sensation in the brain are damaged, causing the transmission of false signals that result in the sensation of pain in a limb or side of the body that has the sensory deficit. The most common of these pain syndromes is called thalamic pain syndrome, which can be difficult to treat even with medications.

The loss of urinary continence is fairly common immediately after a stroke and often results from a combination of sensory and motor deficits. Stroke survivors may lose the ability to sense the need to urinate or the ability to control muscles of the bladder. Some may lack enough mobility to reach a toilet in time. Loss of bowel control or constipation may also occur. Permanent incontinence after a stroke is uncommon, but even a temporary loss of bowel or bladder control can be emotionally difficult for stroke survivors.

Problems Using or Understanding Language (Aphasia)

At least one-fourth of all stroke survivors experience language impairments involving the ability to speak, write, and understand spoken and written language. A stroke-induced injury to any of the brain's language-control centers can severely impair verbal communication. Damage to a language center located on the dominant side of the brain, known as Broca's area, causes expressive aphasia. People with this type of aphasia have difficulty conveying their thoughts through words or writing. They lose the ability to speak the words they are thinking and to put words together in coherent, grammatically correct sentences. In contrast, damage to a language center located in a rear portion of the brain, called Wernicke's area, results in receptive aphasia. People with this condition have difficulty understanding spoken or written language and often have incoherent speech. Although they can form grammatically correct sentences, their utterances are often devoid of meaning. The most severe form of aphasia, global aphasia, is caused by extensive damage to several areas involved in language function. People with global aphasia lose nearly all their linguistic abilities; they can neither understand language nor use it to convey thought. A less severe form of aphasia, called anomic or amnesic aphasia, occurs when there is only a minimal amount of brain damage; its effects are often quite subtle. People with anomic aphasia may simply selectively forget interrelated groups of words, such as the names of people or particular kinds of objects.

Problems with Thinking and Memory

Stroke can cause damage to parts of the brain responsible for memory, learning, and awareness. Stroke survivors may have dramatically shortened attention spans or may experience deficits in short-term memory. Individuals also may lose their ability to make plans, comprehend meaning, learn new tasks, or engage in other complex mental activities. Two fairly common deficits resulting from stroke are anosognosia, an inability to acknowledge the reality of the physical impairments resulting from stroke, and neglect, the loss of the ability to respond to objects or sensory stimuli located on one side of the body (usually the stroke-impaired side). Stroke survivors who develop apraxia lose their ability to plan the steps involved in a complex task and to carry the steps out in the proper sequence. Stroke survivors with apraxia may also have problems following a set of instructions. Apraxia appears to be caused by a disruption of the subtle connections that exist between thought and action.

Emotional Disturbances

Many people who survive a stroke feel fear, anxiety, frustration, anger, sadness, and a sense of grief for their physical and mental losses. These feelings are a natural response to the psychological trauma of stroke. Some emotional disturbances and personality changes are caused by the physical effects of brain damage as well. Clinical depression, which is a sense of hopelessness that disrupts an individual's ability to function, appears to be the emotional disorder most commonly experienced by stroke survivors. Signs of clinical depression include a sense of sadness, sleep disturbances, a radical change in eating patterns that may lead to sudden weight loss or gain, lethargy, social withdrawal, irritability, fatigue or low energy, self-loathing, difficulty in concentrating, and suicidal thoughts. Poststroke depression can be treated with antidepressant medications and psychological counseling.

POSSIBLE TRAUMATIC BRAIN INJURY PROBLEMS

As with a stroke, the severe and some moderate TBI sufferers find that, in a moment, their lives have changed dramatically. The individual goes from being independent to being dependent, from being capable to being less capable. It is compounded by the fact that they cannot even remember the trauma happening. They wake up, and everything is different. What they can remember is being like they used to be: independent, driving, doing things, and going to work. All of a sudden, people are telling them, "You can't do that! You can't get up and walk right now because you'll fall. No, you can't go to the bathroom on your own. No, you can't do this, and no, you can't do that." Anger and frustration are understandable. People with TBI know what they want to do; they can see it, but they can't do it.

In terms of deficits, TBI focuses less on the paralysis and more on cognitive difficulties. Most people with traumatic brain injury, even those that are severe in degree, are walking after their trauma. Within a year, 90% of them get around independently and are able to care for themselves. The cognitive difficulties and behavioral problems have the most significant impact in terms of one's recovery.

TBI has a generalized effect (i.e., the entire brain is affected to some extent). This is different from what occurs with a stroke where a specific hemisphere or section of the brain is affected. With a TBI head injury, there are no, for the most part, patterns of significant deficits in some areas with intact abilities in other areas. Every ability, in a lot of cases, is affected.

Cognitive Skills

Problems that may occur with cognitive skills vary from the very basic arousal or alertness, to sensory and motor skills, to attention and concentration and language skills.

Language-skill problems after TBI may be subtle. An individual may be able to express himself in a basic way but be unable to explain complex things in a logical fashion. One of the more subtle problems that may exist involves word-finding skills. The individual cannot quickly access words from memory. When talking, they tend to talk around the topic. It is difficult for them to "hit the nail on the head." It can be very frustrating finding that correct word.

Spatial and constructional abilities may be affected along with memory. The problem faced by people with TBI is with encoding and retrieving new information. Memory for new information is usually the most severe deficit.

Reasoning skills or the ability to solve may be a problem. Individuals with head injuries often do not recognize the need for a solution or they tend to be inflexible. They may come up with one strategy, but if that does not work, they cannot think of an alternative. They will stick with that same strategy even though it's not working. The basic if-then reasoning that most people use does not occur for these individuals.

Academic abilities are usually not lost; however, the individual may not able to add to their reading, writing, and/or math skills after the injury because of the memory and reasoning difficulties.

Behavioral and Emotional Difficulties

Behavioral and emotional difficulties cannot be separated from the cognitive difficulties that accompany TBI. Ninety-nine times out of a hundred, when there is a behavioral problem, it is tied to a cognitive problem.

Restlessness and agitation are common problems, particularly early in recovery due to the inability to pay attention or difficulties with reasoning. Constant change and irritability are frequently described by families of survivors. When there is damage to the frontal lobes of the brain, the gating mechanism that controls or inhibits actions can be knocked askew such that the person cannot inhibit behavior as well as prior to the injury. The individual is not reasoning effectively and cannot figure out what to do in a situation to solve a problem. To get the attention needed or to generate a response, they may get angry or exhibit other inappropriate behavior. The mechanism that kept behavior under control is knocked askew, and things come out that used to be kept in.

Confabulation is another behavior problem. A patient may tell staff they were at the racetrack for the races last weekend when actually they have been in the hospital for the past two months. The person is not lying; instead, their memory is playing tricks on them. They are not able to organize their memory and, therefore, cannot retrieve information accurately. This person may have been to the track, but in the distant past. Their organizational process, called time-tagging of their memories, is often disrupted and, hence, their inaccurate recall.

Lack of emotional response is demonstrated by a lack of initiative and a flattened affect. The individual does not smile or show any emotional response to things going on in the environment. An example is an adult with TBI who was told by his mother that he cannot drive anymore. His reaction was to put his keys on the dresser and walk out without exhibiting any reaction or emotional response. Most adults would react differently. The emotional response is just not there.

In all cases, it is important to realize that the person to whom the damage has occurred has changed in many significant respects. It is common here at the Stroke Recovery Center to hear loved ones talk about how their significant other has changed—usually not in a positive manner—but rather making his or her care more difficult.

ACUTE REHABILITATION—WHO DOES WHAT?

As long as the patient has insurance of some sort, there is a team of providers that should become involved in recovery at least and until the insurance runs out. The types of professionals who make up the poststroke rehabilitation team consist of the following: physicians; rehabilitation nurses; physical, occupational, recreational, speech-language, and vocational therapists; and mental health professionals. Each may have a part in helping the patient begin the road to recovery and will deal with the various deficits that are the results of the stroke or TBI. For patients that are uninsured, there is a battle to find any help while waiting for help from programs that he/she may become eligible for due to becoming handicapped and/or destitute.

Physicians

Physicians have the primary responsibility for managing and coordinating the care of stroke survivors, including recommending which rehabilitation programs will best address individual needs. Physicians are also responsible for caring for the stroke survivor's general health and providing guidance aimed at preventing a second stroke, such as controlling high blood pressure or diabetes and eliminating risk factors such as cigarette smoking, excessive weight, a high-cholesterol diet, and high alcohol consumption. Neurologists usually lead acute-care stroke teams and direct patient care during hospitalization. They sometimes remain in charge of long-term rehabilitation. However, physicians trained in other specialties often assume responsibility after the acute stage has passed, including physiatrists who specialize in physical medicine and rehabilitation.

Rehabilitation Nurses

Nurses specializing in rehabilitation help survivors relearn how to carry out the basic activities of daily living. They also educate survivors about routine health care, such as how to follow a medication schedule, how to care for the skin, how to manage transfers between a bed and a wheelchair, and how to deal with special needs for people with diabetes. Rehabilitation nurses also work with survivors to reduce risk factors that may lead to a second stroke and provide training for caregivers. Nurses are closely involved in helping stroke survivors manage personal care issues, such as bathing and controlling incontinence. Most stroke survivors regain their ability to maintain continence, often with the help of strategies learned during rehabilitation. These strategies include strengthening pelvic muscles through special exercises and following a timed voiding schedule. If problems with incontinence continue, nurses can help caregivers learn to insert and manage catheters and to take special hygienic measures to prevent other incontinence-related health problems from developing.

Physical Therapists

Physical therapists specialize in treating disabilities related to motor and sensory impairments. They are trained in all aspects of anatomy and physiology related to normal function, with an emphasis on movement. They assess the stroke survivor's strength, endurance, range of motion, gait abnormalities, and sensory deficits to design individualized rehabilitation programs aimed at regaining control over motor functions. Physical therapists help survivors regain the use of stroke-impaired limbs, teach compensatory strategies to reduce the effect of remaining deficits, and establish ongoing exercise programs to help people retain their newly learned skills. Disabled people tend to avoid using impaired limbs, a behavior called learned nonuse.

However, the repetitive use of impaired limbs encourages brain plasticity and helps reduce disabilities.

Strategies used by physical therapists to encourage the use of impaired limbs include selective sensory stimulation, such as tapping or stroking, active and passive range-of-motion exercises, and temporary restraint of healthy limbs while practicing motor tasks. Some physical therapists may use a new technology, transcutaneous electrical nerve stimulation (TENS), that encourages brain reorganization and recovery of function. TENS involves using a small probe that generates an electrical current to stimulate nerve activity in stroke-impaired limbs. In general, physical therapy emphasizes practicing isolated movements, repeatedly changing from one kind of movement to another, and rehearsing complex movements that require a great deal of coordination and balance, such as walking up or down stairs or moving safely between obstacles. People too weak to bear their own weight can still practice repetitive movements during hydrotherapy (in which water provides sensory stimulation as well as weight support) or while being partially supported by a harness. A recent trend in physical therapy emphasizes the effectiveness of engaging in goal-directed activities, such as playing games, to promote coordination. Physical therapists frequently employ selective sensory stimulation to encourage use of impaired limbs and to help survivors with neglect regain awareness of stimuli on the neglected side of the body.

Occupational and Recreational Therapists

Like physical therapists, occupational therapists are concerned with improving motor and sensory abilities. They help survivors relearn skills needed for performing self-directed activities or occupations, such as personal grooming, preparing meals, and housecleaning. Therapists can teach some survivors how to adapt to driving and provide onroad training. They often teach people to divide a complex activity into its component parts, practice each part, and then perform the whole sequence of actions. This strategy can improve coordination and may help people with apraxia (difficulty in structuring thoughts) relearn how to carry out planned actions. Occupational therapists also teach people how to develop compensatory strategies and how to change elements of their environment that limit activities of daily living. For example, people with the use of only one hand can substitute Velcro closures for buttons on clothing. Occupational therapists also help people make changes in their homes to increase safety, remove barriers, and facilitate physical functioning, such as installing grab bars in bathrooms. Recreational therapists help people with a variety of disabilities to develop and use their leisure time to enhance their health, independence, and quality of life.

Speech-Language Pathologists and Therapists

Speech-language pathologists help stroke survivors with aphasia (inability to communicate) relearn how to use language or develop alternative means of communication. They also help people improve their ability to swallow, and they work with patients to develop the problem-solving skills and social skills needed to cope with the aftereffects of a stroke. Many specialized therapeutic techniques have been developed to assist people with aphasia. Some forms of short-term therapy can improve comprehension rapidly. Intensive exercises, such as repeating the therapist's words, practicing following directions, and doing reading or writing exercises form the cornerstone of language rehabilitation. Conversational coaching and rehearsal, as well as the development of prompts or cues to help people remember specific words, are sometimes beneficial. Speech-language pathologists also help stroke survivors develop strategies for circumventing language disabilities. These strategies can include the use of symbol boards or sign language. Recent advances in computer technology have spurred the development of new types of equipment to enhance communication.

It was a speech pathologist that recognized the locked-in syndrome that encased Jean-Dominique Bauby and brought him out of his diving bell and, in his own words, "explains the gratification I feel twice daily when Sandrine knocks, pokes her small chipmunk face through the door, and at once sends all gloomy thoughts packing. The invisible and eternally imprisoning diving bell seems less oppressive." [1]

Speech-language pathologists use noninvasive imaging techniques to study swallowing patterns of stroke survivors and identify the exact source of their impairment. Difficulties with swallowing have many possible causes, including a delayed swallowing reflex, an inability to manipulate food with the tongue, or an inability to detect food remaining lodged in the cheeks after swallowing. When the cause has been pinpointed, speech-language pathologists work with the individual to devise strategies to overcome or minimize the deficit. Sometimes, simply changing body position and improving posture during eating can bring about improvement. The texture of foods can be modified to make swallowing easier; for example, thin liquids, which often cause choking, can be thickened. Changing eating habits by taking small bites and chewing slowly can also help alleviate swallowing problems.

Vocational Therapists

Approximately one-fourth of all strokes occur in people between the ages of forty-five and sixty-five in the civilian population. For most people in this age group, returning to work is a major concern. Vocational therapists perform many of the same functions that ordinary career counselors do. They can help people with residual disabilities identify vocational strengths and develop résumés that highlight those strengths. They also can help identify potential employers, assist in specific job searches, and provide referrals to stroke-vocational rehabilitation agencies. Because of the age group most susceptible to TBI, vocational therapists will be involved in their rehab. Most importantly, vocational therapists educate disabled individuals about their rights and protections as defined by the Americans with Disabilities Act of 1990. This law requires employers to make reasonable accommodations for disabled employees. Vocational therapists frequently act as mediators between employers and employees to negotiate the provision of reasonable accommodations in the workplace.

If covered by insurance, the first stage of rehabilitation usually occurs within the acute-care hospital and may continue at the hospital even when the patient is discharged. Inpatient facilities may be freestanding or part of larger hospital complexes. Patients may stay in the facility for two to three weeks and engage in a coordinated, intensive program of rehabilitation. Such programs often involve at least three hours of active therapy a day, five or six days a week. Inpatient facilities offer a comprehensive range of medical services, including full-time physician supervision and access to the full range of therapists specializing in poststroke rehabilitation.

Outpatient facilities are often part of a larger hospital complex and provide access to physicians and the full range of therapists specializing in stroke rehabilitation. Patients typically spend several hours, often three days each week, at the facility, taking part in coordinated therapy sessions and returning home at night. Comprehensive outpatient facilities frequently offer treatment programs as intense as those of inpatient facilities, but they can also offer less demanding regimens, depending on the patient's physical capacity.

For patients who are not yet able to return to a home environment, rehabilitation nursing facilities may be the next option. They usually place a greater emphasis on rehabilitation, whereas traditional nursing homes emphasize residential care. Fewer hours of therapy are offered compared to outpatient and inpatient rehabilitation units.

Home rehabilitation allows for great flexibility so that patients can tailor their program and follow individual schedules. Stroke survivors may participate in an intensive level of therapy several hours per week or follow a less demanding regimen. These arrangements are often best suited for people who lack transportation or require treatment by only one type of rehabilitation therapist. Patients dependent on Medicare coverage for their rehabilitation must meet Medicare's homebound requirements to qualify for such services; at this time, lack of transportation is not a valid reason for home therapy. The major disadvantage of home-based rehabilitation programs is the lack of specialized equipment. However, undergoing treatment at home gives people the advantage of practicing skills and developing compensatory strategies in the context of their own living environment.

Insurance coverage starts to come into play for those stroke and TBI survivors who do not require institutional help but rather are able to go home. It is not uncommon for benefits for rehabilitation to end in thirty- to ninety days postepisode. It has been the "wisdom" of Medicare that this is the time period in which the greatest amount of recovery will occur, and beyond that time, recovery will be very slow and minimal at best. In order to keep receiving benefits, the patient must be demonstrating measurable progress. At this point, not only do survivors need to focus on getting better but on how to keep the appointments rolling in. Julia Fox Garrison described this problem: "You go through a couple of replacement therapists; you could tell if they were innovative or not and there are times where you feel like saying 'you're just going through the motions.' But you keep it to yourself, because there are times now where you know it won't help your cause to speak your mind. You need each therapist to fight for you—to write letters to doctors and insurers and explain why you need more therapy."[10]

For those with means, this is less of an issue; however, for those who were without coverage before the stroke or TBI or for those who are unable to cover the costs of continued therapy out of pocket, the problems are just starting. Megan Timothy had no coverage before her stroke, and after her emergency treatment and discharge from a rehab facility, she had to fight for coverage. She had a friend to assist her. In her own words: "Jaki's still fighting to get me into Moreno Valley State Hospital for a check up on the effects the anti-seizure medication is having on me. But alas, I've still not been accepted by MediCal and have no money to pay for a visit. I'm stuck hovering in the no-man's-land otherwise known as MediCal-Pending. And my status will remain 'pending' until I'm proven penniless which is far more difficult than you can ever imagine."[11] Megan was poor prior to the episode, but many people who have strokes find themselves unable to go back to work. These survivors have to deplete savings to pay for nursing care or home help. This can lead to forcing a partner or spouse to stop working in order to act as a caregiver. These circumstances can deplete savings as the family tries to cope with the change that the episode has wrought. Therefore, in a relatively short period, families may be finding themselves without the funds needed to continue therapy. Ethnic minorities, Hispanic and African American, have a higher propensity for stroke, which may add to the burden of getting ongoing treatment.

Specifically, in terms of TBI, relatively few individuals receive rehabilitation immediately following their acute medical hospitalization. It is estimated that less than 20% of persons with traumatic brain injury receive acute rehabilitation. Referral to acute rehabilitation is more likely if a physical medicine and rehabilitation physician is consulted, if abnormalities are evident on a CT scan, if the patient is older and unmarried so that there is not much support if they go home, if there are injuries besides the TBI, if medical monitoring is necessary, and if the acute care is lengthy. Recovery is more dependent on what goes on at home and the postacute services that an individual receives.

Caregivers

The individual or groups of concerned family members or friends who care for the stroke survivor need their own systems to support them. Caregivers need to assess their own finances, their confidence to provide care, their means of respite for themselves, and other family support for their work.

ONE OTHER ISSUE

We need to raise the specter of poststroke depression. This is a common complication of stroke observed in around a third of patients where people experience mood disturbances. The mechanisms behind this phenomenon are not well understood, but because it is very common, doctors are usually on the alert for it so they can provide adequate treatment. In addition to depression, people can develop mania or anxiety and other issues.

Some care providers theorize that poststroke depression is caused by functional changes in the brain. According to this theory, people become depressed because their brains are working differently and the balance of neurotransmitters in the brain is disrupted. Other people believe this complication of stroke is a result of stress after stroke. We have seen how stressful and frustrating the deficits are to the stroke survivors. These feelings may be compounded by unhappiness about limited mobility or distress caused by negative interactions with people who are disparaging about the chance of recovery.

The intensity of poststroke depression varies considerably. Some patients experience mild depression and recover as they work through stroke rehabilitation. Other patients start out with stable moods and develop depression, sometimes experiencing a deep depression. Some patients develop major depression. A psychiatric professional can evaluate the patient to learn more about what is happening, to determine how intense the patient's mood disorder is, and to prescribe the appropriate intervention.

Sometimes, simple talk therapy helps a patient with poststroke depression. Patients may find that it helps to stay busy, to interact with friends, and to engage in a variety of activities after a stroke. Regular visits from friends and family may be beneficial, and options like working with a therapy animal, massage, and relaxation programs are also available. For some patients, medications may be necessary to treat the depression, with the doses being adjusted as the patient responds.

Studies on poststroke depression show that it is not something patients can "snap out of" if they are given enough pep talks by the people around them during recovery. Instead, they need to be supported through the depressive episode without being shamed for their lack of energy and pessimistic outlook. If a patient appears to be a danger to himself or others, more aggressive treatment options may need to be pursued for safety.

In the words of one of our survivors: "If you have never had a brain injury or a stroke (and I hope you never have and never will), you'll find that it's virtually impossible to imagine the depth of the injury and the overwhelming fatigue that accompanies it. You can see the obvious disabilities in people who've had strokes or other brain injuries. But what you can't see is the extraordinary effort it takes to do the smallest thing. What you can't see is the way the body responds to the attack on such a fundamental organ. The power of that fatigue is unlike anything I'd ever experienced; there is nothing even close."[10]

"There are many times I thought about giving up. Times when I was too depressed to try… all I wanted to do was put my head under the blanket… and withdraw."[11] The lesson learned is articulated best by Dr. Taylor: "When it came to my rehabilitation, I was ultimately the one in control of the success or failure of those caring for me. It was my decision to show up or not… making the decision to recover was a difficult, complicated and cognitive choice for me."[12]

Depression is also a common problem for individuals after head injuries. The issue is how much of it is organic (related to the brain injury itself) versus reactive to the situation. Fortunately, in either case, the condition is usually responsive to medication and counseling. The danger is that depression can compound the problems that already exist by decreasing activity levels and undermining the expression of skills possessed by the injured person.

The end result for people with TBI and stroke is that they cannot do what they want to do, and they are constantly confronted with frustrations, roadblocks, and hurdles—depression, anxiety, irritation, and bitterness—that can occur after head injury. In the presence of this level of frustration and general distress, it is essential that we focus on the potential improvement in function.

Other potential comorbid or compounding factors include the potential of post-traumatic stress disorder, chronic pain, and substance abuse. Post-traumatic stress disorder symptoms include flashbacks, hypervigilance, nightmares, and others. Chronic pain is the persistent discomfort from an injury. Substance abuse is the use of mood-altering substances to mask the effects of a stroke or TBI. These additional matters should be assessed by a qualified professional as they can abate recovery.

Once that decision to work on recovery has been made, where do you get help?

CHAPTER II

WHERE DO YOU GET HELP?

Help is necessary for recovery. Sources for help become more difficult once insurance coverage has expired. Recovery may take many years, and not only do the survivors see life has changed, but also the families and loved ones find life much different from before the incident. Different loved ones, families, and friends respond to the issues in various manners and, unfortunately, not always in a positive manner. As many stories that we hear of great spouses, wonderful friends, and supportive families, we hear an equal number of stories of abandonment by spouses, families, and friends who are not prepared to deal with the burden of a handicapped survivor. Add that to the financial burden put on the survivor to provide for care, and the challenges to recovery may seem insurmountable. While federal disability is available to those who suffer deficits, the process is long and arduous—can be a two-or-more-year process.

Federal- and state-supported insurance should be available to cover the needed primary care to control the risk factors that may have contributed to the stroke in the first place. While there is little that can be done to reduce the risk of a hemorrhagic stroke, ischemic strokes are subject to numerous controllable risk factors. The strongest precursor to stroke is high blood pressure, controllable with medications. Another controllable risk factor is atrial fibrillation or rapid/irregular heartbeats, also controllable with medications and blood thinners. A heart-healthy lifestyle will help to reduce the risk of stroke: no smoking, moderate use of alcohol, moderate exercise, and weight control. While it may seem that this is closing the gate after the cows have left, recall that the highest risk factor for a stroke is actually having suffered a stroke. Close attention to medications and lifestyles will help reduce the anxiety that is felt by stroke survivors—the fear of that next stroke.

The professional supportive team is the first line of recovery—that is, the physician and team who take care of primary care needs, treat comorbidities (other disease problems), and support general health. Next are the allied health professionals that help with therapies for as long as the insurance continues to pay. Once that coverage ends, we can seek help from families, friends, community resources, and organizations that are focused on stroke and TBI recovery; and of course, if the patient lives in the general area of Palm Springs, California, you can rely on the Stroke Recovery Center for continued help.

FAMILIES AND FRIENDS

While we have many stories of families not willing to accept the burden of a handicapped father, mother, sister, brother, son, or daughter, we have just as many wonderful stories of relatives and friends stepping up and taking a positive role in the survivor's recovery. In some cases, the incident may even make relationships stronger; but in all cases, it changes the relationships that existed in the past.

One of our patients' husbands was a real man's man. In fact, he was on a hunting trip with the boys when his wife had a stroke. He arrived back in town to find her in the hospital unable to walk and unable to speak. Her care fell entirely on him. He retired and accepted his role as caregiver and has said a number of times that it was the best thing that ever happened. He said he never realized how important his wife was to him and how much he loved her. He has rebuilt a van so that he can take her on trips, and they work on her communication skills using computer-assisted means.

Another of our patients' children rejected their mother after her stroke that left her unable to walk, left-sided paralysis, and halting speech. A neighbor in the community they both lived in stepped up and helped, working with her friend to get help first from an assisted-living facility, then from the stroke center, and finally helping her friend to get back home with a live-in caregiver.

While the burden of caregiving falls mainly on spouses (assuming there is one surviving), the network of friends and relatives may suffer a breakdown as those who have surrounded the survivor for years view the patient and understand that the friend, aunt, uncle, or parent is no longer the same person that they knew. There may be the obvious physical disabilities to deal with, but more than that, there may be cognitive problems that are more subtle. Processing of information may take more time and require a high degree of patience that was never needed in the past. Memory issues may affect long-term relationships.

One of the most poignant descriptions of rebuilding relationships comes from Jean-Dominique Bauby, who maintained relationships with friends and relatives through letters and was supported by his wife and children—his mistress (remember, he was French) moved on. As the editor of *Elle*, he was well-known in Paris. "The city, that monster with a hundred mouths and a thousand ears, a monster that knows nothing but says everything, had written me off… 'Did you know the Bauby is now a total vegetable?' said one. 'Yes, I heard. A complete vegetable,' came the reply… I would have to rely on myself if I wanted to prove that my IQ was still higher than a turnip's… Thus was born a collective correspondence… everybody now understands that he can join me in my diving bell… and by a curious reversal, the people who focus most closely on… fundamental questions tend to be the persons I had know only superficially. Their small talk had masked hidden depths."[13]

In her book, *Healing into Possibility*, Alison Bonds Shapiro discusses both the importance and the difficulty of reestablishing a social network of support. "Sometimes people react to brain injuries as if the lack of moving a limb, or the spasticity of walking, means that we're no longer capable of having meaningful social interactions… When my friend Rita went out in public, her disabilities, her halting speech, her unresponsive right arm, and her impaired walking gait caused people to pull away from her… Another stroke survivor, Randy, was very fortunate. His friends at the office knew he needed them. They called. They came by and discussed work problems with him… Sometime the old social body cannot be reclaimed. Then a new one must be built. Providing that opportunity is a vital support that friends and family can bring."[14]

It may be incumbent upon the survivor to redefine the relationships that have existed and to be honest with the needs that now exist. For some, there is a very difficult degree of dependence that did not exist in the past and now must be recognized. But at the same time, there has to be boundaries established to reject enabling behaviors that will not aid in recovery. Julia Fox Garrison stated that she did not want "too much handicapped equipment.... it will sub-consciously send the message that you are planning to remain disabled."[15] Alison Bonds Shapiro related that she had to learn "to ask people to be patient with me because it was important that I be able to tell people when *not* to help me... It's hard for people who love you to watch you struggle. You have to ask for their tolerance."[16]

In the case of TBI, there are some differences because of the focus of cognitive damage to the survivor. However, the provision of support, which in many cases comes from the family, remains the most important factor in recovery. The specific caregiving problems involved in TBI will be discussed in the next chapter.

Friends and family form the front line of support for recovery, but there are other networks of support that will aid in recovery and will also assist the caregiving members of the team. The issues and concerns of caregiving warrant a chapter of their own, but before we look at that, we need to investigate other sources of support that may or may not be available.

COMMUNITY AND ORGANIZATIONS

Dr. Taylor states, "I think it is vitally important that stroke survivors share and communicate about how each of their brains strategized recovery."[17] It is not the community at large but rather the community of survivors that are important to aid in recovery and to share the problems and triumphs. Among the survivors at the Stroke Recovery Center, the consistent theme is the amount of comfort and support they receive from their peer groups. Our patients tell us that their family and friends love them, but they don't understand. We hear that only those who have been through it really know what is happening, and we hear that it is only among peers do people treat you like a whole human being even though you may have deficits. Moving around the Stroke Recovery Center, we see groups that form to work together to help each other, we hear the encouragement in the gym among the groups to keep working on building strength and balance, we hear the group pressure to keep at it and not give in, we see the informal conversations and the formal group meetings, and we recognize the importance of building on the strengths of each other.

While there is no other place in the nation that offers the comprehensive rehabilitation program that is available at the Stroke Recovery Center, there will hopefully be a few options open to survivors in other parts of the country. Because there are estimated to be over 3 million people living with the results of stroke plus an unknown number of TBI suffers, there are support groups that have cropped up in many communities either affiliated with hospitals, medical groups, senior centers, churches, or community centers. At minimum, these provide an outlet to get to know fellow survivors, to share stories and find information to aid in recovery, and perhaps to reinstitute some social life to combat the isolation that can occur.

Overcoming isolation is a major hurdle toward recovery. Julia Fox Garrison stated, "People treat you differently when you are in a wheelchair. In a store, sales people are standing and you're being talked down to. Sometimes they don't even acknowledge you and speak to the person pushing you, as if you're not there."[18] One stroke survivor who was in a wheelchair wrote in one of Stroke Association's magazines that he thought he should become a bank robber because no one ever sees you in a wheelchair. To add to the insult, Julia Fox Garrison asks, "Why do people assume if you are in a wheelchair, you are deaf?"[19]

But it is not only those in wheelchairs who get ignored but also those whose speech is halting, those whose gait is uneven, and those whose thoughts will not come quickly. It is among peers that the survivor can express the frustrations and the triumphs that are all part of recovery. Listening to others' stories and learning from others' experiences all serve as guidelines along the path.

The Internet offers many stories as do the publications of the national organizations that are focused on stroke: the American Heart Association and the National Stroke Association. Both of these organizations have extensive websites that offer resources to aid in recovery along with magazines that relate advances in treatment and stories of survival. The Stroke Recovery

Center website offers links to many resources that are valuable to survivors and caregivers.

The American Heart Association offers programs for stroke survivors that teach people how to play golf. It is important to keep up-to-date on what is being offered regionally and to make the effort to participate whenever possible with those who share the stroke/TBI experience.

The Stroke Recovery Center website also offers access to a virtual clinic. For those survivors who are isolated with no services or groups available in their areas or for those who are not yet able to get outside the house, it provides the opportunity to visit some of the programs we offer here at our facility, along with some educational programs, some therapeutic games and speech assistance programs, and even some light exercise. Also there is the opportunity to interact via e-mail with both our patients and our staff here at the Stroke Recovery Center.

There is a higher level of awareness of TBI because of the number of soldiers who are returning with TBI as well as some noted injuries to celebrities along with the shooting of one of Arizona's members of the House of Representatives. There are proposed TBI centers to help deal with the returning soldiers in California. As awareness of the issue builds, more treatment modalities may become available. Support-group information is available through the Brain Injury Association of America and through the Center for Neuro Skills, both of which are online.

CHAPTER III

CAREGIVERS AND LOVED ONES

Recovery from stroke can be a lengthy process, and the burden of caregiving most likely will fall on the family of the survivor. Caregiving is a burden no matter how willing and able the loved one is to assume the new role. Along with the emotional toll, financial stress may add to the problem; and because of the probable long-term need, the issues may get worse over time. In the case of those with means, there may be the ability to hire a professional caregiver for full-time or part-time help to allow for greater freedom of the family caregiver, but in most cases, this is not an option.

While we often think of caregiving as being a one-way relationship, caregiving involves a partnership between the patient and the caregiver. Each member of the partnership has his or her own problems to deal with, not only coping with the situation, but also helping the patient to thrive. There is a responsibility on the part of the patient along with problems unique to caregivers. These issues and problems are common to all caregivers, and a frank and open discussion should be part of the recovery process; however, it is often necessary to have a third party facilitate these discussions and help to define the roles of each of the players. While we concentrate on groups for the survivors at the Stroke Recovery Center, we also provide groups for the caregivers, both family and professional. In needed cases, we will facilitate one-on-one discussions and help to find solutions to problems. In the following sections, we will examine the problems that exist between the patient and the caregiver as well as the problems that are just the caregivers.

CAREGIVERS AND PATIENTS

A difficult factor for the caregiver to recognize is the change in the loved one beyond the obvious physical deficits. As put by Dr. Taylor, "Although I looked the same and would eventually walk and talk the same as I did before the stroke, my brain wiring was different now, as were many of my interests, likes and dislikes… From the beginning it was vitally important that my caregivers permit me the freedom to let go of my past accomplishments so I could identify new areas of interest. I need people to love me—not for the person I had been, but for who I might now become."[20]

As stroke survivors, Alison Bonds Shapiro states, "We have a responsibility to our caregivers as well as to ourselves. Our job is to ask for what we need and make clear what we don't need at the same time we find ways to care for, appreciate and be patient with our caregivers. They love us. They're doing the best they can with a job that they're not prepared for, in a situation that causes them to struggle with their own emotions."[21] Dr. Taylor delineates her needs: "I need my caregivers to teach me with patience… When people raised their voices while teaching me, I tended to shut down. I was essential that my caregivers remember that I was not deaf; my brain was simply wounded… I need people to come close and not be afraid of me. I desperately needed their kindness. I needed to be touched—stroke my arm, hold my hand, or gently wipe my face if I'm drooling."[22]

Professional caregivers, from physicians to home health aides, have a tendency to objectify patients. Typically, the health practitioner treats diseases rather than individuals. This expresses itself in talking about the patient as if he or she is not there, addressing the loved one instead of the patient, treating the disease, not the person, and generally marginalizing the humanity of the survivor. While it may seem in some cases that the person is not aware, remembering the case of Jean-Dominique Bauby's locked-in syndrome should give us all cause to look at all patients as individuals with feelings, thoughts, imagination, humor, sexuality, and hopes and aspirations. Eye contact, physical contact, reassurances for however small the achievement, and recognition of the person beyond the disease is critical to the patient's recovery. The stroke survivor needs to know they still have value and that their dreams are achievable.

Professional caregivers and family caregivers share a common problem of enablement. A part of this is the willingness and wanting to help your loved one or your patient that is at the basis of the profession of health care. However, the ability to do even the simplest things on one's own helps to form the basis for regaining some control over one's body and one's life. Julia Fox Garrison shares an experience with her husband, Jim: "You are in the bathroom, and you are standing there in the dark. You make a promise to yourself: 'I am not going to the bathroom until I can turn on the lights in here.' You have been struggling with it for several minutes when Jim happens to walk past you in the hallway. He flicks the switch without missing a beat."[23] It is difficult to watch someone you care for struggle. Caregivers must show the patience and tolerance to allow the survivor to triumph over what they may view as the smallest things and allow for the time for the survivor to formulate thoughts, words, and actions.

Socialization—the development of new friends and groups of people who understand and relate to the problems both the patient and the caregiver are going through can be very helpful to the process. Never underestimate the healing power of laughter and fun. It is an important part of regaining control over one's life and one's facilities. Julia Fox Garrison wrote a list of dos and don'ts for doctors, but they are every bit as applicable for caregivers: "Lead patients without using murky medical jargon; Inspire your patients to create their own goals; See the unique characteristics of each patient; Enable your patients to feel safe and confident; Provide positive words of hope, courage and support; Treat the mind as well as the body. Above all, listen."[24] As one of our patients at the Stroke Recovery Center stated, "You can talk to your family and you know they love you, but they just don't understand." She feels that the ability to be a part of the community of caring that we nurture here at the center was instrumental in her regaining her ability to walk, drive her car, and resume much of her life prior to her stroke. Caregiving can sometimes mean being able to let go and allowing the patient to build relationships of help themselves in a safe and comfortable environment.

The ability to listen is the major factor in expressing the needed patience. We hear over and over that family members rush patients. Finishing the patient's sentences, rushing the thoughts, moving on before the patient has a chance to formulate his thoughts and make a cogent response, and being confused when a number of things are being thrown at them are all complaints we hear. It took Jill Bolte Taylor eight years to get back to teaching—recovery is a slow process.

In the case of TBI, there are some differences. Severe TBI in particular presents families with a tremendous burden because of the cognitive and behavioral problems that people with TBI exhibit: irritability, memory problems, and reasoning difficulties. Since TBI sufferers tend to be younger in most cases, the parents (particularly mothers) fulfill the role of caregiver. TBI survivors may require constant supervision of a professional caregiver as well.

CAREGIVING PROBLEMS OF FAMILIES AND LOVED ONES

There is no way to minimize the difficulty, the stress, and the problems that informal or family caregivers have to confront. During any given year, there are more than 44 million Americans—21% of the population—who provide unpaid care to an elderly or disabled person eighteen years of age or older. Most caregivers, 61%, are women, middle aged, and employed. More than half of employed women caregivers have had to make changes at work, such as going in late, leaving early, or working fewer hours.

One of our survivors writes, "The role of a caregiver is really very difficult. Caregiving requires you to show up and be helpful at the same time you're dealing with your grief and rage that someone you love is suffering. Caregiving thrusts a responsibility into the midst of your life that you may be unprepared for, and you may have little time or resources with which to meet that responsibility."[25]

In 2006, *Journal of Gerontological Nursing* published a study from Northwestern University regarding caregiving for stroke survivors. Of great interest were the causative factors of stress, which will be discussed in detail. Most studies in the past have focused on the care of Alzheimer patients that have related depression and stress among caregivers to increased mortality. On the other hand, this study indicates that apart from the strain of the situation itself, the primary caregiver of a stroke survivor suffers the most stress from unhelpful family members. It is the lack of understanding and tangible help from friends and relatives that is responsible for the most depression and anxiety.

The details of the study, along with a review of the existing literature, were designed to identify the most difficult times, unmet needs of caregivers and advice for the first two years of caregiving, and perceptions of the importance of resources used and not used. Research in the past has revealed three classes of stressors that were most disturbing: stroke-related, living environment, and the caregiver's physical and psychological well-being. Being confined to home and having little time to themselves are both reported as problematic for new caregivers. The most difficult problems were the stroke survivor's emotions, negativity, noncompliance, and care-related interpersonal issues. Need for information on recovery expectations, preventing a recurring stroke, and managing role changes along with counseling and skill training have all been identified as needed to reduce the problems of caregiving.

Seventy-six percent (76%) of caregivers in the study identified the hospitalization and/or the first two months at home as the most difficult time. The distressing factors included uncertainty, new responsibilities, lack of support, and the survivor's impairments and emotions. One respondent stated, "I was helpless, scared." Another stated, "I didn't have confidence. I was afraid of doing something wrong and worried about another stroke." Later, the comments shift toward concern for a plateau of functions: survivor and caregiver health problems, finances, and the caregiver's emotions. Added to this may be the stress of balancing work. One husband commented, "I have no help and have to keep a job… I can't do anything for pleasure." As the years go on, concerns for legal assistance and life planning emerge.

In terms of unmet needs, three themes were predominant. Feeling unprepared was very common in the first months. Enhancing the survivor's emotional and physical function and sustaining the self and the family emerged later. The effects of chronic caregiving can be noted in the following comment: "Now is the most difficult time because I am tired of being a caregiver, drained physically and mentally. The first year was physically the hardest, [there was] more uncertainty and he was able to do less. But now, it is the tiredness of the whole situation." And with the long-term burnout and frustration comes guilt for feeling these negative thoughts.

On the other hand, from the point of view of the needs of the patient, the caregiver role, to be most effective, has to be very engaged and very active. What is meant by this is that the stroke survivor requires socialization, stimulation, reintegration into society, and activities using the brain and the body. It is unfortunate that we see time after time at the Stroke Recovery Center that family and/or friends are unable or unwilling to provide this active caregiving function to the survivor. It is an all-consuming job and can be a frustrating job as healing is a slow process. Seeking help and assistance from organizations, professional caregiving services, day-care services, and helpful friends can alleviate some of the pressure that falls on the loved one.

With TBI, as mentioned before, the likelihood of the burden of caregiving will fall on the family. Families are also rightly concerned about the future needs of their injured family member. Parents, being older, are more likely to pass away before the injured person. So there is a concern about who is going to take care of their child if he or she needs long-term care.

At the Stroke Recovery Center, support groups for the caregivers have equal importance to those for the survivors. In some cases, it is of value to have the caregiver and survivor meet together. In some cases, it is of value to have the caregivers meet with other caregivers and compare problems, coping mechanisms and methods of relieving stress, and resources that can aid in the care. As one of our family caregivers said, it is good to have someone to cry with. If the survivor has high-enough functioning, the Stroke Recovery Center may offer respite for the caregiver who can drop off the loved one and have some time to him or herself. Numbers of our family members will volunteer in another part of the center while the survivor is doing therapy. This is a good distraction and offers interactions for the caregiver with others who are not caregivers while at the same time they are close at hand and can see their loved one forming friendships and gaining back some of the control over his or her own life. Local resources that can offer this type of intervention have demonstrated that combining survivors and caregivers in the same group can lead to further understanding and support. Recently, a caregiver spoke of the anger directed at her by the stroke survivor. Another survivor was instrumental in educating that caregiver to the feelings and stressors he felt. That exchange between two strangers proved strengthening to the caregiver.

Health of the caregiver is very important. The anger of the survivor and the burden of ongoing care put severe stress on the caregiver. We have seen a number of our family caregivers break down physically and emotionally. It is important to be able to leave the loved one without feeling guilt, being comfortable that the survivor is being cared for—even if it is only for an hour or two. On the other hand, there is joy to caregiving. Getting to know your family member at a different level than ever before and being able to give off yourself to bring joy and comfort to others. Giving instead of taking, helping others who are unable to help themselves, and putting someone else first are all rewarding in and of themselves.

The words of one of our valued volunteers at the Stroke Recovery Center and the leader of our counseling programs, Lois H. Kahn-Feurer, PhD, writes, "As a severe TBI survivor I am aware that I could not be at the level of rehabilitation I have achieved with first the medical care I received in seven weeks of hospitalization and the ongoing care and support I receive from family and friends. Let me add that like so many other survivors, I have experienced one family member who has abandoned me since the accident. Others have remained strong, enduring and persistent in their love and care. Today, my recovery is considered miraculous as I returned to full time work, driving my car, walking without assistance and teaching. I would not complete an intelligence test while in the hospital for fear I would be embarrassed by the results. I persistently belittled the activities lead by the physical therapist for fear I could not complete them. As part of my current work, two years after leaving one of the hospitals in which I was a patient I returned to give a talk. I apologized to the staff if I had offended any of them while I was a patient. Afterward, one of the staff said he appreciated my apology and 'yes, I was the patient from hell' as I had described myself. My recovery is today supported by the Stroke Recovery Center where I volunteer. There I am among fellow survivors who understand that while many of us bear no visible signs of our brain injury, the psychological and emotional scars are still there. Scabs over these scars prevent constant fresh injury. Gratitude provides additional strength. Newcomers to the Center remind us all where we have been and hopefully provide a road map for ongoing recovery."

CHAPTER IV

STROKE RECOVERY CENTER OPTIONS

In many cases, the system is stacked against recovery for stroke survivors. It is the "common" wisdom among the medical profession that recovery of function occurs in the first few months following the stroke. Beyond that time, achievement of gains is considered to be negligible. Because of this, the insurance industry, taking its lead from Medicare, tends to only allow for a very limited number of physical therapy and/or speech therapy visits and no payments for any type of recreational therapy. For those without the resources to pay for therapies, options to continue improving may be nonexistent.

The Stroke Recovery Center offers the stroke survivor the options of continuing exercise therapy, speech therapy, and recreational therapies designed to challenge the cognitive issues involved in recovery. *All services are free.* We understand that only a very small number of people who need services are in our area and able to physically join us, so we are trying to put more services online to help more people. We have proven over the years that recovery keeps on for a number of years, and survivors must never give in or give up.

LET'S TALK RESEARCH

Our research has shown remarkable results over the three-year periods that we have been tracking outcomes. The methodology is to gather data regarding outcomes of treatment for chronic stroke and TBI sufferers from the existing patient base and compare such data to stroke and TBI victims and survivors along with national data regarding seniors and disabled populations.

In the most recent year, we collected and tabulated data for 89 clients who, as of January 1, 2009, were Stroke Recovery Center users, having been there 3+ months and attended at least 3 times per month or more. We were able to compare the data points with the cohorts we collected in years 1 and 2.

The initial baseline data was analyzed using the criteria of length of attendance (LOS) at the Stroke Recovery Center. Looking at the year 3 data, we found that the length of attendance remained a median of 2 years with the heaviest concentration continuing to be in the 2- and 3-year time frame consistent with the year 1 and 2 data. Having three years of data, we were able to track the dropout rate and analyze the characteristics of those who do not continue and reasons for noncompliance with the program along with the utilization criteria we determined in the year 1 and 2 study.

With the median LOS at 2 years, data points were again compared to determine if there were differences in the early users as compared to those who have been at the center for 2+ years. With that data in hand, analysis went deeper to look at the changes from year 1 and 2 as well.

The data findings were addressed and compared to data from year 1 and 2 in the following categories:

Client Dropout in Year 2: This category was identified as clients who had attended at least 3 months in 2009 and had dropped out by December of 2009. There was an 11.2% dropout as a percentage of the whole. However, of that number, 44.6% were from death and/or deteriorating health issues that no longer allowed the client to participate at the center. The other reasons reported were moving out of the area, return to work, and no reason.

Age and Sex of Clients: The average age of clients is 68.8, similar to the first year of the study. The median age is 69, slightly lower than year 2. As expected, the group that has a longer LOS (length of stay) has a slightly higher average age of 71.8. The client base continues to reflect national norms with the highest propensity for stroke being in the 60–79 age group and men and women being at equal risk.

As the group ages, men become higher risk; but prior to 60 years of age, women have almost twice the risk over men. This is supported by our sex differentials that show a higher propensity of women in the first 2 years with the men catching up as the LOS extends.

Prescription Drug Usage: Prescription drug usage per patient increased to 7 per patient in year 3. This is in line with the Kaiser study of seniors that identified 7 medications as the norm. Examination of the drugs indicates a wide variety of drugs used, including dietary supplements and vitamins. Comorbidities appear to be the major determining factor and suggest that drug usage needs to be examined on a case-by-case basis.

Transportation: The shift to public and/or commercial forms of transportation and a return to self-transportation continue to support that rehabilitation efforts increase confidence and independence and decrease reliance on family. Professional caregivers as transporters remain constant. Bus usage moved from 5.3% in the first 2 years to 20% in the over-2-years group.

Ambulation: Year 3 data indicates that there is a continued aggressive move to utilize mobility aids among the patients. Initial data seemed to indicate that there would be less use of support aids as the years went on; however, the data suggests the opposite is true. Stability and balance are critical to successful mobility and independence. The use of aids appears to enhance that process.

Orthotics: Initially, it was contended that orthotic use would decline as the years progress, but as with ambulation aid, the use of orthotics has increased as the years progress. This suggests that orthotics use is being prescribed to increase balance and mobility in an aggressive manner and should be correlated to reduction in falls.

Emergency Room Visits: In 2009, 17.3% of the patients made at least one visit to an emergency room (ER), even less than the prior years. All these visits came from the group who has been at the Center less than 2 years.

As the patients remain at the Center, the propensity to use the ER declines, which offers significant savings to the health-care system.

Falls: The percentage of patients who fall has declined each year of the study to 13.5% in year 3. This number is well below the national average for seniors of 30%. The increased use of ambulation aids and orthotics can be correlated to this as the concentration on balance and strengthening use individually in the exercise therapy program can be cited as supporting these numbers.

The research that we have done clearly demonstrates the benefits of long-term rehabilitation in not only bending the quality of care curve, but also bending the cost curve to long-term care. We shall go into this in more detail in the last section of this book as we examine the cost benefits to providing long-term rehabilitation to the health-care system as a whole.

For years we have been a singular voice, promoting the benefits of long-term rehabilitation with very little support from either the academic or the medical profession. However, Dr. Pamela W. Duncan (principal investigator of the Locomotor Experience Applied Post-Stroke [LEAPS] trial and professor at Duke University School of Medicine in Durham, North Carolina), along with her colleagues, presented findings on 11 February at the American Stroke Association's International Stroke Conference 2011 in Los Angeles and also on February 12 at the American Physical Therapy Association's (APTA) 2011 Combined Sections Meeting in New Orleans. Both presentations support the benefits of low-tech continued rehabilitation.

The study found that patients continued to improve up to twelve months after suffering a stroke, defying the widely held view that recovery happens early and peaks at six months. In fact, this study showed that even patients who started intensive rehab six months after a stroke improved their walking.

Stroke patients who had intensive home-based physical therapy improved their walking ability just as well as those who underwent a more high-tech program. This approach of locomotor training included settings where they walked on treadmills with their body weight supported by a harness. The results of this study showed that more expensive, high-tech therapy was not superior to intensive home strength and balance training, but both were better than lower-intensity physical therapy.

For the study, they recruited 408 patients of average age 62 who recently suffered a stroke and were being treated at six stroke rehabilitation centers in the United States between April 2006 and June 2009. The participants were 45% female, 58% Caucasian, 22% African American, and 13% Asian. They were assigned to have 36 sessions lasting 75 to 90 minutes for 12 to 16 weeks, either completing the locomotor training (starting at two or six months after stroke) or the home-based training (starting at two months after stroke). In all three groups, the program was structured and progressive, and the patients had to achieve specific goals and tasks.

The home-based program, which started at two months after stroke, aimed to improve patients' strength, balance, flexibility, and range of motion as a way to improve walking. The main measure the researchers were interested in was how much each of the three groups' walking had improved one year after stroke. However, they also looked at what it was like at six months after stroke.

The researchers' assumption at the start of the study was that by the end of the twelve-month study period, the patients on the more high-tech locomotor programs would show better improvements than the ones on the home-based exercise programs, especially the ones that started their locomotor training two months after stroke.

But what they found was the following:

- After twelve months, all groups made similar gains in walking speed, movement or motor recovery, balance, social participation, and quality of life.
- 52% of all participants had made significant improvements in their walking ability.
- The timing of the locomotor training did not make a difference; after twelve months, there were no differences between the early and late locomotor-training groups in terms of the proportion of patients who improved their walking ability.
- Stroke severity did not affect their ability make progress by the twelve-month mark.

In all groups, the biggest improvements in outcomes were made after the first 12 sessions of therapy, but 13% of the subjects continued to make functional gains in walking recovery by 24 sessions and another 7% improved by 30 to 36 sessions. There were some differences between the locomotor and home-based groups in that patients in the locomotor groups were more likely to feel dizzy and faint during their exercise and those in the early locomotor group had more falls. Also, 57% of all participants fell once, 34% fell more than once, and 6% had a fall that resulted in injury.

At the Stroke Recovery Center, we have found that the benefits of exercise continue in the strengthening and the balancing of the survivors and are particularly important in relieving the problem of falls. With the presentation of this research, we hope to see follow-up that may help to support the work we do here and encourage long-term rehab availability elsewhere.

SUCCESS FACTORS

Functions compromised when a specific region of the brain is damaged by stroke can sometimes be taken over by other parts of the brain. This ability to adapt and change is known as plasticity. "I needed people around me to believe in the plasticity of my brain and its ability to grow, learn and recover. Overcoming negativity is a major hurdle to recovery." Dr. Taylor continues, "I have heard doctors say, 'If you don't have your abilities back by six months after your stroke, then you won't get them back!'... this is not true. (she) noticed significant improvement in (her) brain's ability to learn and function for eight full years post-stroke, at which point (she) decided her mind and body were fully recovered."[26] Dr. Kahn-Feurer continues to note marked improvement from her TBI since 2002. She has, for example, greater strength and accuracy in her golf game and walks generally with more balance and strength. When one day complaining about her golf game, a peer reminded Lois, "When you first came on the course, we were amazed you could stand after striking the ball. You have come a long way." Cognitively, Lois notes increased memory function. Other survivors relate the same type of experiences from doctors, therapists, and other professionals promoting acceptance of the disability and adaptive behavior to deal with the deficit when what you want to do is get better.

The attitudes of the survivors and those that surround the patient have an immeasurable effect on the recovery process. It is important to focus on the abilities and not the disabilities, to build on what one can do, to celebrate the triumphs (those small miracles) however small. Goals should be lofty with achievable steps along the road supporting hope. While strokes are serious business, we cannot negate the power of fun in the recovery process. Finding pleasure in one's life helps to minimize the inevitable stress that will arise.

How to maintain the motivation, the positive attitude, and the will to keep striving to improve is a major hurdle to recovery. In many cases, the patient may be undergoing shifts in how thoughts are processed, emotions that, in their prior life, were either nonexistent or much easier to control. Patients that were used to being independent now find themselves dependent upon someone else for many of the ordinary activities of daily living. And to add to these not inconsiderable problems, the patient may have to deal with an outside world that is not handicapped friendly. Although the ADA rules have made mobility easier and have increased access, there is a long way to go in changing attitudes toward the handicapped. We have a tendency to warehouse those among us who are not whole either mentally or physically, to ignore or even shun those who suffer a handicap, forgetting or ignoring the human being that is within the shell however battered it may appear. As a survivor or as a caregiver to a survivor, this makes motivation and optimism even more difficult. For example, our own international airport does not provide ramps to access planes unless requested in place of drop-down stairs. Rather, staff will offer to lift the disabled individual to the plane. Searching through the literature for long-term recovery of functionality results in a lack of support for continued hope. While most experts agree that there will be spontaneous recovery of some functionality in the first three months following the incident, there is little to no agreement for a continuing road map for recovery of further functionality. The importance of the paper delivered in February 2011 at the Stroke conference in Los Angeles, California, that we cited earlier in the chapter may well be the first paper that supports continuation of rehabilitation beyond those first few months. However, from the point of view of the last thirty-two years of rehabilitation that has been provided at the Stroke Recovery Center, the study does not go nearly far enough. As a start though, it does encourage the use of low-tech exercise to promote continued improvement. We promote at the Stroke Recovery Center focusing on getting better rather than just getting used to one's disability.

An element that is missing in the study and one that we believe to be a critical success factor in recovery is the availability to and the building of a community of support for the patient. In many cases and well documented among those who have written about their strokes, the group of friends and family, even those who remain very supportive, have little understanding of what the survivor is going through. In many cases, the survivor may feel very differently, may have problems relating, and may show different personality traits as the brain heals. The ability to form a community of survivors, to discuss the incident with those who have experienced brain damage, to discuss issues with a peer group—things like "Is it safe to have sex again?" "How do I get my family to slow down around me?" "Living with the fear of having another stroke"—issues that can best be discussed with those who have gone through the same fears, anxieties, and depressions.

The study emphasizes the importance of ongoing exercise to recovery, a stance that we support 100 percent at the Stroke Recovery Center. Two additional things that we must add are that exercise can continue to aid in recovery well beyond the additional six months, the study documents, and once again, we contend that the development of a support group adds to the benefit and will result in greater functional recovery. Not to discount the benefit of home-exercise programs since, in most cases, this will be all that is available to the survivor, the additional stimulation and support that is found in group exercise or inclusion in a gym setting promotes recovery to a higher level as we have documented in our research. While it is difficult, if not impossible, for stroke survivors who suffer from physical deficiencies to exercise at community gyms, a setting that is devoted to stroke and TBI survivors introduces the same camaraderie and group support that one enjoys at a regular gym. There is the element of competition, the element of cajoling, and the element of delight for the achievements of one's friends that cannot be achieved at home.

In a book by Norman Doidge, MD, featured on PBS's *The Brain Fitness Program*, he talks about patients who have continued to improve three years after their strokes. He states, "Because it is a use-it-or-lose-it brain, we might assume that the key areas of (the)... brain for balance, walking, and hand use would have completely faded away, so that further treatment would be pointless. Though they did fade, (the) brain, given the appropriate input, was able to reorganize itself and find a new way to perform the lost functions—as we can now confirm with brain scans."[27] Efforts in retaining the speech of patients who averaged 8.3 years from their last stroke showed that 30% had a demonstrated increase in communication capabilities. While the doctor is promoting the benefit of constraint-induced therapy, we have had similarly remarkable results in speech pathology at the Stroke Recovery Center, even as long as ten years poststroke.

Stimulation, rebuilding of confidence, taking part in the community are all important in continued recovery. In most areas of the country, there will be at least a support group of stroke survivors that discusses many of the problems and triumphs that are shared in this community. There are also a number of magazines that focus on stroke put out by both the National Stroke Association and the American Stroke Association that are available for all. The Stroke Recovery Center offers online support through our virtual clinic where a survivor can join in some of the programs we offer and participate in our community. All these things will help to keep the patient stimulated and engaged in his or her recovery. The process can be very slow, which only means that engagement is critical to the long-term health of the survivor.

An important point to keep emphasizing in long-term treatment is the element of stimulation. Be it in exercises, meals, or activities, routine can very quickly devolve to boredom. There is a fascinating ongoing experiment in senior long-term care that is being conducted by the Eden Alternative. This organization is forming senior communities based on the principles of eliminating loneliness, helplessness, and boredom. While not dealing specifically with stroke or TBI populations, the principles are applicable. What they have discovered in building their communities, routine needs to be broken with variety in activities, meals, and day-to-day necessities to alleviate boredom. They have also documented great benefit in introducing levels of responsibility among their residents dependent upon ability, from the caring for a plant to the caring for a pet. Visit www.edenalt.org for more information on this interesting organization. While options like the Stroke Recovery Center, whose principles follow the same lines as the Eden

Alternative, may not be readily available, the concepts can be integrated into the recovery program of each individual.

One further issue that needs attention is the importance of diet. Because of the imposed immobility and, for some, the loss of functionality, it is easy to see a gain in weight. Attention should be paid to providing a heart-healthy menu, teaching and coaching how to provide meals for oneself that are healthy and nutritious, cooking with one hand, using the microwave, avoiding burning oneself on the stove—all things that able-bodied persons take for granted. At the Stroke Recovery Center, we invite patients to join a heart-healthy lunch every day. There is an additional benefit to this in that we are retaining and encouraging the patient to eat in public. There are products that assist those who have limited use of hands and arms to help cut food and to assist in eating that we introduce if needed. We encourage the patients who can to eat and drink with others while enjoying a social meal.

While strokes and TBIs are very serious businesses, it is very important not to forget to laugh and have some fun. If we invest too much seriousness in the process of therapy and recovery, we miss a big part of what's life-giving and important. If we are miserable, we focus on our losses rather than focusing on our strengths. At the Stroke Recovery Center, we mix entertainment and fun, including monthly outings to the movies, the art museum, the casino, and/or other venues with our therapies. We understand the value of fun.

The issue of payment is a significant deterrent to the expansion of stroke recovery centers throughout the nation. All our services are free, and as mentioned, there is no federal, state, or local reimbursement available. Because of this, no insurance companies offer payment even as an option to long-term survivors. At the Stroke Recovery Center, 80% of the patients are of middle to low and very low income. The patients come from all walks of life with the only common denominator being the stroke or TBI. The intent of the free service is to eliminate any barrier to recovery due to cost and to reduce any differences or class systems that may result from the ability to buy particular services in the center. This is an important tenet to our treatment and the philosophy of the Stroke Recovery Center.

CHAPTER V

ALTERNATIVE THERAPIES

The American Stroke Association and the National Stroke Association each put out a monthly magazine that we mentioned as a resource for ideas for rehabilitation. Along with articles, there are numerous ads directed to stroke survivors. These ads make all types of claims and promises to help speed recovery. We will go over a few of the alternative therapies that we have identified. But as a word of caution, we advise that one asks your physician, physical therapist, speech therapist, or some other professional before embarking on a course of treatment. While we introduce alternative therapies at the Stroke Recovery Center, we do not endorse any of the programs offering devices or supplements. For those programs that involve the patients physically, we have the patient's physician sign a release stating the patient can tolerate the therapy.

Although there is a body of knowledge that states acupuncture is ineffective in the treatment of stroke, we have introduced it as an alternative treatment modality at the Stroke Recovery Center. Julia Fox Garrison talked about acupuncture: "For acupuncture treatment to work, you have to put your mind into it as well as your body... you have to let the world stop and concentrate on the healing process... you quickly learn that you cannot go one time and expect a miracle."[28] We will be tracking the effectiveness of the acupuncture on relieving spasticity in the hand over time and are hoping to discover an effective treatment methodology over time and attempt to show improvement in flexibility and use of the fingers. The numbers involved in our case studies will be small due to the time limits and the total number of patients who are eligible for the tests; however, if the results are positive, we will hope to have further studies done on a larger scale to demonstrate efficacy.

One of the survivors who participates at the Stroke Recovery Center has written three books about her recovery, including the time she has spent with us. Madelina Agawin is a strong believer in natural medicine, and in her book, *The Healing Fields,* she discusses dietary supplements, massage therapy, the use of magnets, and hypnotism as alternate therapies that she believes in and has used to some effectiveness over the period of her recovery. Madelina addresses her peers at the center on a regular basis and, along with a strict vegetarian diet, seems to be a good model for her method of recovery.

We regularly offer yoga and tai chi as low-impact alternatives for exercise. These can be done from wheelchairs as well as from upright positions and seem to aid in balance and some gentle strengthening. Stretching and relaxation are some things that most can participate in no matter how severe the deficiency.

Some of the most effective therapy aids are in the speech therapy area. Computer-assisted communication devices are available to help aphasic survivors. Available in both laptop and handheld versions, the devices can help the patient formulate sentences and communicate wants, needs, and desires. Most of these aids are reimbursable by insurance.

There are numerous other types of alternative therapies that people will defend, including the use of a synthetic form of Indian curry and the use of magnetic pulses to stimulate the brain, to name just a couple.

We are firm believers that any and all therapies require application and patience for lasting results. Alternative therapies should be checked out with your primary physician to make sure they will do no harm. Cost factors should also be taken into the mix; some of the therapies that have been demonstrated to our patients are not reimbursable by insurance, which means there may be a significant out-of-pocket expense. As mentioned, we at the Stroke Recovery Center believe very strongly in the benefits of exercise, speech, and recreational therapies and are slow to suggest alternative therapies.

That said, the next section will be devoted to the Stroke Recovery Center—what we do, our philosophy, our treatments, funding, and building a board of directors—all that is needed to set up a stroke recovery center in another area.

SECTION II

THE STROKE RECOVERY CENTER

CHAPTER I

HISTORY

The Stroke Recovery Center is a nonclinical, inexpensive combination of programs that offer long-term rehabilitation to the survivors of stroke along with support for their families, caregivers, and loved ones. The Stroke Recovery Center is unique in that it provides comprehensive services at no cost to the stroke survivor or his/her family. Being ineligible for health insurance reimbursement, the Stroke Recovery Center welcomes patients whose health benefits have expired and provides services as an adjunct to services the survivor may be eligible for under his or her insurance plan. Since the majority of patients are with us for years rather than months and, as noted, recovery may take many years, there are few patients who have remaining visits with therapists. Additionally, it is of note that recreational therapies are not reimbursed by insurance carriers. In some states, adult day-care services are funded, and they may include some recreational therapies, but comprehensive therapeutics, such as those presented at the Stroke Recovery Center, fall outside the norm for inclusion in adult day-care centers, senior centers, and/or nursing homes.

Over thirty-two years ago, Dr. Irving Hirshleifer started working with stroke survivors and their families to provide stimulation and some limited therapies designed to aid in recovery. Using an initial $10,000 donation, he created the Palm Springs Stroke Activity Center and began the arduous task of raising money to help this underserved group of survivors. Programs and numbers expanded from a small dedicated group to a comprehensive program when generous donors purchased a 17,000-square-foot building and donated it for our use. With the support of a dedicated board of directors, the center was able to survive its founder's death and continues to thrive to this day. Changing the name of the organization to the Stroke Recovery Center to emphasize the concentration on recovery and carving out seven thousand square feet to set up a thrift shop set up the center to continue its work to the current time.

Having collected years of anecdotal results (miracle after miracle) in 2007, we instituted tracking systems and collected data to support the premise that our therapies resulted in both a bend in the quality curve and a bend in the cost curve in terms of long-term provision of care in chronic disease. The center was named for best practice in long-term care by the California Heart Disease and Stroke Prevention and Treatment Task Force (Department of Health Services) in *California's Master Plan for Heart Disease and Stroke Prevention and Treatment 2007–2015*.

Programs were developed from evidence-based programs that were cited in the literature as well as from identified need. The physical component of recovery shifted from a physical-therapy model to an exercise-therapy model and introduced more in the way of low-impact therapy, massage, and personal training. Computer-assisted speech instruments were introduced to aid in the treatment of aphasia, Wii therapy was added for coordination and competition, and in 2011, a virtual clinic component was added via the web for those unable to come directly to the center.

The center has served as a model for the development of services in a number of cases, but other programs have been unable to raise the funds needed to provide services for free or have been unable to provide the full spectrum of services, leaving the Stroke Recovery Center as a unique entity in the country. Having an operational budget of approximately $700,000, the center relies exclusively on fund-raising events, foundation and family donations, and revenues from its thrift shop to fund the services it provides to over 260 clients per year, five days per week, on an outpatient basis.

CHAPTER II

PHILOSOPHY

The Stroke Recovery Center focuses on treatment of the whole person, offering a safe environment with respect given to each client and his/her family and loved ones. Staff and volunteers work with each patient, recognizing the humanity within each regardless of the severity of their impairment. The center works with the imagination, the humor, the anger, the depression, and the sexuality of each patient, along with the specific physical, cognitive, and communication disorders that may exist. The philosophy of the center focuses on treatment of the mind, the body, and the spirit, challenging the physical, the aesthetic, and the mental capabilities of each of the patients combined with social interaction and just plain fun.

Developing the trust to give the patient and the families the confidence of safety and security forms the basis for successful recovery. Careful selection and training of the staff is critical to assisting the improvement in mind and body that we have documented over the years. All members of the staff must be able to see beyond the handicap and work with the patient as an individual. They must be trained to help but not do—let the patients develop the skills of doing daily tasks no matter how long it takes. The staff is also trained to listen rather than talk and to try to bring out the positive in each and every patient.

There are many sensitivities that we are cognizant of and work hard to overcome. We encourage a supportive touch to the arm or shoulder of a patient, we encourage competition among patients, we encourage free expression of opinions and views, and we are very sensitive to loss and shared grief for our members, volunteers, and caregivers who have died. At the same time, we have to adhere to a line between staff functions and support and the caregiver and/or the social worker support systems that may be needed for the patients to thrive. We have resources we can refer the patients and the families to, but we cannot fulfill all the needed functions internally. What is meant by this includes functions such as driving patients to appointments, loaning or giving money, and socializing with or giving shelter to needy patients. Because of the close nature of the relationship between therapists and patients, the staff becomes very attached, and the loss of patients is traumatic to both staff and clients. We encourage unscripted grieving circles that include both staff and volunteers and families of the departed that allow for open discussion of the person, their foibles, and our relationship to them. We shed tears together and laugh together as an extended family. It is this type of environment that supports the maximum long-term recovery and is imperative to replicate to achieve consistent results.

Additionally, there are nuances that are very important in developing and adhering to our culture. To support the safe and secure environment, we must be egalitarian. The defining differences in our clients are the stroke or TBI and the damage that has resulted. This is one of the strongest reasons that our services are free and, even though there are great difficulties in raising the necessary monies for upkeep of the building and staffing, the board of directors and the management have never wavered in their commitment to keeping the services free. While we ask for a membership fee of $25 per year if the patient and family can afford it, there is no privilege to be gained by joining, only a sense of pride in being able to help. It is important to not introduce a structured approach to services. Stroke and TBI survivors have, in all likelihood, issues with insurers before they have arrived on our doorstep, and it is our job to dispel those anxieties and concentrate on healing. While a full 20% of our patient base would, in all probability, be able to pay for services, we would not like to see a stratified society develop at the Stroke Recovery Center based on ability to pay. The lack of uniforms, lab coats, and/or formal business attire among the staff helps to dispel the distance between the staff and the patients. The focus is on making the patient feel like a part of society again.

Using a significant number of volunteers allows the center to present programs that would otherwise be out of range from a budgetary perspective. While many of the volunteers who work in the kitchen and the thrift shop are retired, there are many active volunteers who give up time at the office or from busy practices to spend a few hours a week or a month with the patients either teaching skills, educating, or entertaining. Volunteers undergo the same training in relationships as the staff, understanding the need to work with the patients as individuals while not enabling physical and cognitive handicaps. The sixty to eighty volunteers that work provide more than 16,500 hours of service yearly.

Maintaining a positive environment for healing—understanding the seriousness of stroke and TBI but not being overwhelmed by it—is what makes the Stroke Recovery Center as successful as it is.

CHAPTER III

PROGRAMS AND SERVICES PROVIDED

The center offers exercise therapy focusing on balance and strengthening of the weak side, with both individual and group treatments. Speech therapy is offered on an individual and group basis along with computer-assisted communication therapy using both individual programs and computers designed to assist communication. Recreational therapists offer a schedule of activities to fill the day. These programs vary from rap sessions on current events, group sessions dealing with recovery issues, word power, improvisational theater, life-coaching discussion groups, arts and crafts, computer usage and Wii to entertainment and bingo. The programs are designed to promote interaction and peer-support development along with cognitive improvement. A healthy-heart menu is offered every day for lunch along with an early morning light breakfast and coffee time. The charge for this lunch is $3, the only service that requires payment.

EXERCISE THERAPY

Through long-term and consistent exercise therapy, patients will achieve their maximum potential for recovery from stroke and TBI symptoms. Focus is on correcting poststroke balance problems and on strengthening of limbs weakened or paralyzed by the stroke. Toning up the cardiovascular system to increase general health is also stressed.

After being evaluated for admission to the Stroke Recovery Center, if exercise is appropriate for the patient, he or she must collect a medical release from their doctor stating that they are able to tolerate exercise. (We additionally require a medical release for acupuncture.) The admission procedure allows us to gather information that can then be tracked on a yearly basis to monitor the effectiveness of our programs. We may determine that a caregiver's presence is necessary to ensure the safety and security of the patient. At the exercise room's initial visit, the patient's special needs for therapy are identified by the patient and the exercise therapist in a one-on-one meeting. A therapeutic exercise regime is created to meet the needs of the individual patient. Following that, the patient may arrive on any day, Monday through Friday, between 8:30 AM and 12:30 PM (exercise therapy room hours), and use the equipment. An appointment is required for a thirty-minute (30) private session with the fitness trainer. These sessions are a part of therapy and not for single use.

Therapists measure patient progress by comparing their current physical status to that of the start of therapy. The patient and therapist work together to identify progress made, set new goals, and make progressive changes and extensions in the exercise routine. Progress notes and reviews are done on regular bases that change according to the initial goals that the patient and the therapist have worked out in the initial visit. Lofty goals are encouraged, but all goals are admirable as research has shown even low-intensity exercise will help in recovery. Blood pressures are taken at the center for the initial visit and upon request.

The following is a list of some of the equipment used in the gym:

MOTOmed. A motor-assisted movement therapy system for arm and leg therapy. Level of difficulty can be adjusted to suit the patient's needs. A computerized system provides data on efficacy of patient's work. It measures the amount of effort the patient puts forth, the synchronicity of limb movement, and the duration of the exercise. The MOTOmed strengthens weak muscles of arms and legs. This machine is adaptable for leg and arm exercises.

Parallel bars. Two bars parallel to each other in an upright position approximately thirty-nine (39") inches from the platform. Provides safety for gait training, balance, and strengthening exercises. A full-length mirror in front of the bars allows patients to see themselves and check their body position.

Recumbent bicycles. Recumbent bikes offer the opportunity for leg strengthening. Patients are able to move onto the bikes using the swivel seat and position legs on the pedals with straps to hold them and allow for both downward and upward pressure.

Nonweight pulleys. The patient controls a rope on a pulley with his hands and arms to stretch to maximum highs and lows. This improves range of motion, prevents frozen shoulder, and helps prevent or correct subluxation. The patient is encouraged to gradually increase the range of stretching while not having any discomfort. A holding mitt is used to hold handles when patients are unable to maintain a grip.

Weighted pulleys. Used to develop upper-body strength and coordination. Weights are adjustable, and handles can be pulled from low, middle, or high positions. This works the different arm muscle groups. A holding mitt is used on hands that cannot grip the handles.

Arm turntable. A horizontal, flat, round table with a handgrip and forearm support. The patient rotates the circle using the affected arm. Rotation circles can be adjusted from small to full extension. This enhances the patient's range of motion and coordination of elbow and shoulder.

Bayou fitness leg trainer. A glide board to lie on while using legs to push the body back and forth. The body weight is used as resistance (i.e., exercising directly against the body weight). Slant degree can be adjusted according to patient's ability. This is also a very good exercise to correct foot drop.

Cybex abdominal crunch. A chair where the patient sits with hands attached to weighted straps that are pulled forward and released backward using the abdominal muscles only. Strengthens abdominal muscles as in sit-up exercises.

NK leg lifts. A large chair with hinged leg lifts. At the side of these lifts, various weights are placed to adjust levels of difficulty. For quadriceps strengthening, patient rests feet under a pad on the leg lifts, then lifts and holds legs upward. For hamstring strengthening, the leg lift is raised, and the patient pulls downward with his leg.

Fine-motor hand exercises. A table containing various small objects used to strengthen and develop coordination of hands. Examples are the following: transferring golf balls to an empty basket, putting pegs in holes, and using button and zipper closures.

SPEECH AND LANGUAGE THERAPY

Many stroke survivors are affected with expressive or receptive speech disorders. These difficulties may range from serious problems, such as total inability to express oneself, to minor problems, like a slight slur. A speech and language pathologist evaluates each patient for speech problems and then assigns a plan for each patient to follow. Most problems require one-on-one therapy; however, where appropriate, group sessions are invoked. Volunteers are used to assist patients in the group settings.

Expressive speech is evaluated beginning with simple yes-and-no questions and moving on to identifying places or things. For patients unable to speak at all, a computer program may be appropriate or a simple communication board can be used in identifying important things in the patient's life.

Receptive language skills involve work on sequencing speech. This is taking the patient from a one-step command to a multiple-step command as the patient progresses.

Reading skills are also part of speech therapy, and if there are no visual problems involved, volunteers often work with patients on reading. Choosing age-appropriate reading material and a subject that the patient finds interesting is important. Reading material may include the following: newspapers, magazines, books, or articles. It is important to not use children's books or magazines unless the patient is a child. As with all the therapies, it is important to allow the patient to make mistakes and self-correct. Assessment is made as to the receptive ability of reading online as well as by holding a book, magazine, or newspaper. Some clients have noted they are better able to comprehend using one of these methods over the other.

Handwriting is also part of speech therapy. Patients often have to relearn to write using the unaffected hand. Handwriting is taught by beginning with the basics used in grammar school and progressing as fine-motor control is regained to writing names and short sentences.

It is of interest to note that within the patient base of the Stroke Recovery Center are numerous persons who have communication difficulties but do not choose to participate in speech therapy. Some have developed finely tuned systems of communication using limited verbal and body language to express needs and wants. While we try to encourage verbal communication, we adapt to meet the needs of the individual patients as well. It is interesting to note as well that we have numerous patients who have little to no English language skills. While the majority of these are Spanish speaking, we have two that speak eastern European dialects. We have Spanish-speaking staff available to handle issues but encourage the Latino group to participate with the non-Latino group and find that they work out a communication system to meet the needs of each of the participants.

RECREATIONAL THERAPY

There are a great many elements that go into recreational therapy. While many senior and care centers will default to activities directors, the Stroke Recovery Center is committed to licensed recreational therapists as the leaders and developers of the structured programs that are designed to encourage cognitive healing, some physical healing, and emotional and social development. The emphasis is on therapeutic activities rather than just activities to provide distractions. Retraining of the mind along with retaining the body requires a strict adherence to therapeutic discipline without putting an onerous burden on the patient. In other words, it is the skill of the therapists that combines the retraining with the proper amount of socialization and entertainment that helps to build the community and develop the skills needed for recovery. Every month, a full program calendar (see calendar in appendix) is delivered to the patients, posted in the center, and put on the web page. Patients and caregivers are encouraged to join in on whichever activities they choose. However, all are encouraged to join the life-coaching sessions for patients, for caregivers, and for families to help deal with the emotional problems that confront all the survivor community.

There are many different types of activities that can encourage recovery. Some examples are the following:

Rap Sessions

The purpose of the rap sessions is to encourage communication and interaction between patients and the volunteer or staff member in charge of this session. The emphasis is on communication skills, socialization skills, and memory skills.

Topics for the rap session should not be offensive to individuals and should be age appropriate. Talking about controversial subjects, such as religion or politics, requires strong leadership skills as discussions can get contentious and active. The patients will come from diverse cultural, ethnic, and economic backgrounds, making for lively and interesting groups.

Topics for rap sessions may include the following:

- current events (local, national, or worldwide)
- current television programs (*American Idol*, the Academy Awards, etc.)
- fashion (what people were wearing at an event, what is popular in fashion)
- foods (favorite foods, restaurants, diets, etc.)
- music (favorite music, popular songs, etc.)
- pets (pets they have had throughout their lives or a pet they now have)
- science (something currently happening in the scientific world)
- sports (championships or regular games)
- upcoming holiday (individual traditions, what people are doing, etc.)
- vacations (where are they going, what are they planning on doing during vacation)

Speakers

Subject matter experts are invited to speak about a variety of subjects, basically, anything that may spark patient interest or add to the client's knowledge base to help manage their health and welfare.

Possible topics may include the following:
- dietician: heart and stroke healthy diets
- expert on current events: health-care issues
- doctors, nurses, or other medical professionals who have a specific expertise
- medical insurance advocacy groups: HICAP, etc.
- pharmacist: drug interactions with foods, etc.
- local transportation
- travel (with photographs)
- environment: local animals, plants, terrain

One caveat on bringing in experts is that they, the speakers, are not allowed to sell the patients anything. A number of these experts will have a book, a product or products, or a service that they are promoting. It is made very clear that any attempt to solicit extra business will result in immediate ejection.

Music/Entertainers

Musicians and entertainers are brought in on a regular schedule as well as for special events. All types of music are appropriate if they appeal to the broad audience. Entertainers such as dancers, comedians, and/or magicians may be invited to perform. Youth groups as well as adults are welcome.

Music and Dance

Persons with brain damage from stroke or traumatic brain injury have been shown to exhibit significant improvement as a result of music therapy. This is theorized to be partially the result of the synchronization of movement with the rhythm of the music. Consistent practice leads to gains in motor skills, cognitive processes, and language skills.

Brain function physically changes in response to music. The rhythm can guide the body into breathing in slower, deeper patterns that have a calming effect. Heart rate and blood pressure are also responsive to the types of music that are listened to. The speed of the heartbeat tends to speed or slow depending on the volume and speed of the auditory stimulus. Louder and faster noises tend to raise both heart rate and blood pressure; slower, softer, and more regular tones produce the opposite result. Music can also relieve muscle tension and improve motor skills. It is often used to help rebuild physical patterning skills. Levels of endorphins (natural pain relievers) are increased while listening to music, and levels of stress hormones are decreased. This latter effect may partially explain the ability of music to improve immune function. A 1993 study at Michigan State University showed that even fifteen minutes of exposure to music could increase interleukin levels, a consequence that also heightens immunity. Literature has also shown that the brain can relearn with rhythm and lyric while language development remains slow.

Comedians

Laughter is the best medicine. Research has shown that laughter increases the secretion of the natural chemicals (catecholamines and endorphins) that make people feel good. It also decreases cortesol secretion and lowers the sedimentation rate, which implies a stimulated immune response.

Oxygenation of the blood increases, and residual air in the lungs decreases. Heart rate initially speeds up and blood pressure rises, then the arteries relax, causing heart rate and blood pressure to lower. Skin temperature rises as a result of increased peripheral circulation. In addition, laughter has superb muscle relaxant qualities. Physiologists have shown that anxiety and muscle relaxation cannot occur at the same time and that the relaxation response after a hearty laugh can last up to forty-five minutes.

While stroke and TBI are serious, it is important to build in laughter and joy to aid the healing process.

Games

There are many types of games, including board games, card games, puzzles (crossword puzzles, sudoku, cryptograms, jigsaw puzzles, logic problems, and word-search puzzles), memory games, physical games, and Wii games. Many games provide a social context where socialization takes place along with the game itself. Most games also provide many benefits that the individual may not realize are occurring (e.g., playing cards is excellent for increasing fine-motor skills). Increased memory is a factor in all games that involve thinking, and it has been proven that if the mind is utilized, the individual cognitive abilities will remain.

The following are some of the different types of games and their benefits whether played on computer or in person:

- Board games, card games, and puzzles improve hand-eye coordination, sequencing, number identification, color identification, fine-motor skills, logic skills, memory skills, and socialization skills.

- Cards and jigsaw puzzles are excellent for increasing fine-motor skills, and if the individual utilizes the weak hand during the activity, it will improve fine-motor dexterity. Many skills are taking place to improve the patient's abilities simultaneously while the patient is focused on socialization.

- Memory games may include games such as Jeopardy!, 21 Questions, and Trivia, among others. These games help stimulate the memory and help provide logic and socialization skills.

- Physical games may include games such as boccie, bowling, golf putting, parachute games, shuffleboard, and volleyball. The goal is to increase one's individual abilities and not the competitive goal of winning or topping another individual. The games stimulate increased range of motion, increased strength and endurance, increased hand-eye coordination, and in many cases, increased fine-motor skills.

- Wii games are excellent for increasing fine-motor skills, range of motion, hand-eye coordination, memory sequencing, logic skills, color identification, and number identification, as well as introducing a healthy individual and team approach to competition.

Arts and Crafts

There are many different types of arts and crafts projects: acrylic painting, beadwork, ceramics, collage, craft projects, etching, needlework, oil painting, paper mache, scrapbooking, watercolors, and woodworking.

For the individual stroke survivor, a stroke may leave them suffering with emotional, psychological, and adjustment issues as a result of the impact of the trauma on their physical and cognitive functioning.

Coping strategies, memory, learning skills, the ability to think or organize thoughts, emotional reactions, behavior, social interactions, relationships, communication, language, and understanding can all be affected. Because of this, the habits and skills developed to cope with trauma or change—to plan and live life—can no longer be relied upon in the same way, often leaving the person feeling confused, alone, unable to communicate, anxious, and depressed.

Art as a form of therapy is particularly helpful for people who find it difficult to communicate verbally, have survived trauma, or who are facing times of adjustment and change. An image or colors or textures can express complex thoughts and feelings that cannot be made sense of or put into words. As an unconscious form of communication, the images made are seen and understood alongside and with the patient. For stroke survivors who may have been catapulted back to a state of helplessness and dependence and a world without words or meaning, this creative space is one that holds the potential for the following: self-expression and nonverbal communication; the containment of feelings; and for finding form, color, texture, and meaning to the physical and psychological experience of stroke. Through absorption in the art-making process within the frame of the therapeutic environment, the individual may then begin to regain a sense of their capacity to combine thought and physical action.

Art as therapy may increase abilities for expressing thoughts and feelings that may not have words, leading to greater understanding and awareness, more meaningful communication, and a decrease in anxiety and depression by channeling emotional and physical energies in constructive and potentially coherent manners, leading to a more flexible exploration of possibilities and resulting in more adaptive responses to life's challenges. Art as therapy can lead to the mastering of anxieties and may contribute to feelings of control, dignity, empowerment, and independence.

These are few of the types of programs that are offered under the RT umbrella. Other ongoing programs include access to and instruction in the computer lab. Patients are encouraged to use the Internet along with playing games online. Additionally, there are speech programs available for the patients to work on their own. Large screens for the vision impaired are provided as well.

THE FOOD PROGRAM

The food program has two different parts: early morning coffee and Continental breakfast and, at 12:30 PM, full lunch. The morning coffee and rolls are available for all patients and caregivers to start their day after they sign in. Breakfast-type foods are offered, such as fresh fruits, English muffins, bagels, toast, muffins, coffee, teas, and juices. The morning offering is designed to give the patients the opportunity to gather in a social setting for conversation and camaraderie. Patients are encouraged to prepare their own beverages and snacks, giving them independence and skill development. Volunteers are on hand to assist for those requiring additional help. Patients can also be seen assisting each other—another benefit of this morning routine.

Lunch is designed to provide a nutritious and healthy meal. This is often the main meal of the day for many of the patients. Menu planning is done on a six-week rotational basis, altering days for each menu item to reduce predictability so that those patients who have regular days would not receive the same meal every time they attend (see menus in appendix). Additionally, the menus are revised on an as-needed basis dependent upon coordination of food donations from community food banks and retail organizations throughout the local region. Preparation of food is done in a healthy manner with a balance of vegetables, protein, and starches. There is very little fried food served, and fat and carbohydrates and salt are kept to a minimum. Soups and salads are made with fresh produce as available from local sources, and fresh herbs and selected seasonings are used to provide savory flavors without the use of sodium. Portion control is an important factor in our menu planning.

Special menus are prepared for holiday events and special celebrations. The dining area is decorated in themes for all holidays, and the food is planned to meet the occasion—turkey for Thanksgiving, hot dogs (appropriately prepared to prevent swallowing difficulties) for Fourth of July. Festive and fun attitudes prevail with all services done by volunteers aided by staff when needed. The staff and volunteers are encouraged to eat with the patients and the caregivers.

CHAPTER IV

WHAT IS NEEDED FOR A STROKE RECOVERY CENTER?

PATIENTS

The very first thing that is needed for a Stroke Recovery Center is patients. In eastern Riverside County, California, where the Stroke Recovery Center is located, a health assessment done in 2009 (HARC) estimated there are fifteen thousand stroke survivors alone. This says nothing of TBI survivors. Ask in a group of people who knows a stroke survivor, and you will find it is unusual to not have a show of one or two hands even in very small groups. But the challenge is how to get those people to the center and engage in the recovery process. Referral sources include the local hospital's stroke programs, the rehabilitation departments, local physical therapists, and local speech therapists. Each of these professionals have motivation to work in concert with the Stroke Recovery Center because the center acts as a continuation of care for the patients when there is no more money available for professional billing. It means that the professional does not have to totally abandon the patient to his or her own treatment but rather act as a conduit to the next level of care. This whole process and what it means to a stroke recovery center will be more clearly defined and discussed in the advocacy section of this book.

Other sources of patients may not be as obvious: community centers, assisted-living centers, skilled nursing homes, rehabilitation homes, senior centers, service clubs, churches, mosques, and synagogues—in other words, anywhere groups of people congregate. In these areas, there may be stroke and TBI survivors, friends, and/or family members who need the services of the center. These people are reached by a strong outreach program that consists of public speaking, attendance at health fairs, and constant discussion on the local media to raise awareness of the problems of stroke and TBI and the availability of hope.

PHYSICAL NEEDS

With patients to serve, the next issue is a physical space and the equipment needed to provide the comprehensive programming. A stroke recovery center can be initiated in limited space, bringing in food and drinks and carefully organizing programming. However, to function at the higher level, the physical space should include a gym, a kitchen, and an activities space along with office spaces, specialty rooms for arts and crafts, computers, meetings, speech therapy—individual and group, plus reception. Approximately seven thousand to ten thousand square feet is adequate space to run a program. Once the space is committed to, there is the need for equipment for the gym, to the kitchen equipment, to recreational-support equipment, to tables and chairs for activities, to meals, to meeting rooms and offices. Computers and software to support a small business are also needed for bookkeeping and record keeping as well as communication and research. The space needs to be cheery, accessible, and attractive to support the feelings of hope and health.

STAFFING

Delineating the needs and identifying the programs and services that are necessary to providing comprehensive programming clearly make the staffing roster become evident. There are two different components to the management of the program overall: first is the hands-on therapy plus general operations, and second are the development functions: outreach, volunteer coordination including board development, and fund-raising. At the Stroke Recovery Center, we resolve the financial constraints by combining full- and part-time positions with contract workers to keep the budget manageable and staff at a minimal number. Current staffing is at 8.5 FTEs with fourteen employees.

CONSTRAINTS

Once the capital needs for a center are met, the biggest challenge is to build and attract ongoing operating capital. Developing and adhering to a strict budget is critical for success. While health care attracts a significant amount of charitable giving among higher-income givers, it is necessary for organizations to prove their value to donors: individuals, foundations, trusts, and public funders. Proving value means that outcomes must be positive, documented, and replicable, not just anecdotal. The Stroke Recovery Center has developed the model for success and has also developed the systems needed to track and report outcomes that support the continuation of the program by showing its value to both the quality and cost curves of the health-care system as a whole. The system begins with the evaluation of patients before being admitted to the program. While entrance requirements are not stringent, we do not accept the dual diagnosis of dementia or Alzheimer's with stroke and/or TBI. The reason for this is that we cannot provide the one-on-one attention needed for this type of disease. Additionally, we require a full-time caregiver for those patients unable to toilet or feed themselves. In our intake process, we ask a commanding list of questions: demographic, medical history, family situation, and utilization of services. It is from this intake process we are able to design a program for the individual patient and to initiate the process with the center. While progress is tracked in the gym and in specific programs such as acupuncture, we have a yearly review of the patient's progress in relationship to his or her ability to deal with activities of daily living and within the parameters that are delineated in our ongoing research (research in appendix). Having been able to demonstrate success longitudinally gives us a positive, provable, and fundable story for funders to feel comfortable in supporting.

One other system that is critical to success is the audit trail. What is meant by this is funders need to see that their charitable dollars are being appropriately spent on the programs and services that go to the needy population, not the board of directors, chief executive officer and directors, or even the staff. As a 501(c)3 corporation, there is a public trust factor that is important to success. With thirty-two years of history as of 2010, the Stroke Recovery Center has credible systems in place to make funders comfortable, to attract new donors, and to provide a credible partner in the development of continuum of care services for the provision of long-term and chronic care. The Stroke Recovery Center has manual personnel, operations, and financial management. Each of these elements is a factor in raising the ongoing funds needed for operations. Development or fund-raising has a number of elements and is worthy of its own segment.

DEVELOPMENT: RAISING MONEY

The Stroke Recovery Center is currently entirely dependent upon fund-raising for its operational budget commitment. There are three major sources of ongoing funds: individual contributions, grants, and special events. Once one has discounted the patient base as no more than a token source of funds, all efforts go toward maximizing the other sources.

Grants are a specialized form of giving and require a very detailed level of attention. They can cover the spectrum from pages of detailed input required to a single sheet of information about the organization. Grants can come from small family trusts, city or other public sources, large specialized foundations, and/or community foundations. A level of expertise is required to maximize the effectiveness of solicitation. Data, both operational and financial, is required for submission, and the utilization of money received must be tracked and reported upon. The quality of the submission and the data tracking has great influence on the continued support from the grantor. For this reason, the Stroke Recovery Center has developed systems for tracking daily usage of each program: duplicated and unduplicated numbers, volunteer hours and numbers, new client evaluations, demographics—age, income, sex, and home location (see tracking report examples in appendix), along with the financial tracking systems needed for monthly reporting to funders and the board of directors.

Special events make up an important part of any fund-raising mix. Events can vary from major galas to spaghetti dinners to golf tournaments to walks to fashion shows. The purpose is to raise awareness for the organization, to involve as many different demographics as possible, and of course, to raise as much money as possible.

Donor development and special-event planning and follow-through are full-time jobs requiring community involvement and social networking at the highest-level charitable givers. The highest levels of the organization—director of development, CEO, and the board of directors—all need to be involved in the efforts to develop the contacts, to build awareness, and to form communities of givers who will attract other donors in an expanding circle of influence among charitable donors in the community. The credibility of the organization rests on the presentation made to the public, and all care needs to be taken to present the organization in a positive and attractive manner.

Raising the capital to start a stroke recovery center has its own issues and challenges. There may be funders in the area who can be educated to the value of having the Stroke Recovery Center as a resource to reduce the burden of long-term costs that chronic disease puts on providers. Beyond that, there may be donors who have a particular interest in stroke and/or TBI and are willing to donate to build a center. Additionally, there may be empty municipal or county buildings that would be suitable for conversion and available at little or no cost. All these avenues must be searched down and, if possible, exploited to raise the capital to get a stroke recovery center started.

Recognizing the difficulty of dependency on fund-raising, it is important to understand how health-care reform will affect the creation of comprehensive care models that can and should include stroke recovery centers. Additionally, opportunities to generate alternate revenues from services that are provided should be explored. An example of this is meal services that could be provided for homebound programs (such as meals-on-wheels), or space rental to outside groups for meetings or for fund-raising for other organizations, or collaborative efforts with other organizations to share services and revenues. Analysis of assets that are currently available and opportunities to leverage those assets is the first step to sustainability. Ideally, the Stroke Recovery Center of the future will have a base of predictable funding and will be able to use fund-raising to supplement project development and special needs.

THE IMPORTANCE OF LEADERSHIP: BUILDING A BOARD

The experience of the Stroke Recovery Center has proven that there are two separate and distinct functions that need to be addressed in order to build a successful center. While the center attempted to manage both functions under one umbrella, the difficulties have resulted into a bifurcation of functions into two distinct 501(c)3 organizations, each with a different mission and goal and different boards of directors with differing skills and backgrounds.

The initial organization holds the operations and includes all patient care, equipment, and staff. This organization focuses on quality of care issues, building patient bases, developing relationships with existing health-care providers, attracting and training volunteers, and taking care of the building. In the case of the Stroke Recovery Center in Palm Springs, this also includes a thrift store that is located on-site, but this service is site specific and not a necessary adjunct to the overall services and programs. The management of this organization focuses on the personnel, the clinical provision of services, and the financial management of the operation. Operational maintenance and management are under this organization and include things like the groundskeeping, utilities, insurance, and grant expense. The type of board member who is most valuable to this organization will have expertise in rehabilitation at some level, health-care provider credibility to develop need contacts for referrals, fiscal management expertise to help in budget development, and financial management and/or personnel experience to aid in attraction and retention of staff.

The second organization is a fund-raising organization led by the senior management of the organization and staffed by the development staff. Bookkeeping, reception, and general secretarial functions can be shared. This board of directors should be filled by prominent members of the community. As many of the board as possible should also be major donors themselves. This adds to the credibility of the organization and to the ability to bring in other major donors. Major functions should be chaired by prominent donors who can bring in not only their friends but also other prominent donors in the community. A bonus is that the more prominent members of the community also attract media coverage and add to the general appeal of your charity. People love to be associated with a winner.

Senior management must have the ability to span both organizations, which means not only the understanding of both the health-care issues that the organization confronts but also the social and charitable organization issues that come to the fore. Ideally, the leader should have strong presentation skills and the ability to motivate staff, along with in-depth knowledge of the financing and working of the health-care industry. The leader should have the ability to develop and communicate a strategic vision relevant to both boards and be able to produce credible budgets to support the goals. Most importantly, the leader must have the ability to work with the foundation board, building a strong and consistent donor base that can be counted on year after year.

CHAPTER V

BARRIERS TO DEVELOPMENT

There are two significant barriers to the development of stroke recovery centers built on the successful model we have presented: expertise and money. The easiest barrier to overcome is the development of expertise since the model exists, has been tested, and is both efficient and effective as long as the appropriate level of money can be raised. That, of course, raises itself as the major barrier and is the explanation for why there is only one stroke recovery center in the country that offers a comprehensive program for free. Not only is that a barrier for starting a stroke recovery center, but it is also a barrier that must be confronted year after year. Once the capital expenditures to get underway are covered, the core operations must be covered and cash flow for payroll and ongoing expenses accounted for and budgeted so that short-term borrowing is not needed for continuing expenses. Small organizations have little in terms of cash reserves to fall back on, so the challenge of short-term management is considerable.

It is important to understand the financial barriers in some detail.

CATCH 22 FOR CBOS

Sustainability is the key for the long-term survival of CBOs (community-based organizations) like the Stroke Recovery Center. The center can provide services at a relatively low cost because it has flexibility in staffing, use of volunteers, and is not forced to provide clinical services and food services that are regulated by various agencies of the state and/or federal government. However, therein lays the catch-22. Because the center is a nonclinical and unregulated provider of care, there is no public agency that oversees its operation, and therefore, there is no agency that provides funding for the services and programs. Further, since there is no public agency under which the organization falls, private funders of health care, namely health insurance companies, follow suit and do not fund these organizations either.

The cost benefit to the health-care system as a whole as reflected in the research is enhanced because of the low cost of the service provision. The low cost cannot be sustained under current possible government reimbursement scenarios.

GOVERNMENT AND/OR PUBLIC FINANCING

The complexity of the financing of health-care services in the United States make it exceptionally difficult for community-based organizations to find a niche in which to carve out the few dollars that are required to provide their wealth or health benefits. The Stroke Recovery Center benefits the survivor and the families; the economics of which will be detailed in the next section of this book. However, the center does not offer a direct benefit to outpatient rehabilitation centers. Since there is no reimbursement for chronic care, survivors are not offered services; and since rehab is not provided as an emergency, there is no charitable care imperative. As a point of explanation, if, for example, an uninsured patient requires emergency care in an ER, the physicians and the hospital are bound by law to provide the emergent care. That bill is then written off as charity care. Long-term or chronic care is not an emergency, so it would never fall into this scenario.

On the other hand, benefits may accrue to the funders of inpatient rehabilitation and skilled nursing facilities in the long-term because of the ability of the Stroke Recovery Center to allow patients to live in their homes and be supported by their families. The high cost of institutionalization falls on state and federal government providers and is a major cause of health-care inflation.

Most stroke survivors will qualify for health-care coverage under the American Disabilities Act, although the process is arduous and very frustrating. That said, physician and hospital visits will be covered; however, since this is a high-risk group, the ability to keep them in the community and out of the hospital can have a positive effect on controlling health-care costs as a whole. One of the ways that the government is attempting to help control costs and change the reimbursement incentives to keep patients out of the hospitals is to impose a strict fine on hospitals for readmissions in under thirty days. This is an area where the Stroke Recovery Center can assist the hospitals, having proven its ability to keep the patients out of the hospitals and to reduce falls.

Many hospitals are seeking accreditation for stroke treatment to enhance the quality of care given at the acute level. The accrediting organization is called the Joint Commission on Accreditation of Healthcare Organizations or JCAHO. When a hospital wants to become an accredited stroke center, it must provide physician coverage, nursing expertise, appropriate protocols for treatment, and also long-term care plans. It is this area that may offer opportunities for stroke recovery centers to partner with local hospitals as a low-cost provider of continuing care for stroke patients. Additionally, if reimbursement incentives follow the track as proposed in the Affordable Care Act to include continuing care, there may be extra money available to allow for a carve-out payment for organizations that are providing low-cost, long-term care. Understanding the various models and the role of advocacy that is needed will help to ensure that this population is no longer allowed to fall through the safety net.

SECTION III

ADVOCACY

Stroke and TBI are serious businesses. The fact that the need for long-term care is not currently met by our medical community places a burden on the families and the survivors that can result in the breakdown of the family fabric as well as the health and well-being of the survivor and those that surround him/her. This in turn may result in additional burdens on society in terms of increasing health-care costs. Although a difficult road, advocacy is needed at all levels, from the community to the federal government. Education is needed to make those who control the purse strings aware of the pervasive nature of the problem and the effect on society that the current lack of resources for this population has on our financial health as a nation. To be an effective advocate, it is important to understand the economics of stroke and the costs to society as a whole as well as to understand how each and every individual can act as his or her own advocate at all levels. Additionally, an understanding of the demonstration models of care that are being funded and examined under the proposed health-care reform is helpful in building a consensus to support inclusion of the care of this disadvantaged population.

ECONOMICS OF STROKE RECOVERY

Estimates of the yearly costs of stroke vary from $43 billion to $73.7 billion. These numbers include the direct cost of care, which include hospitalization, physician fees, rehabilitation, and medications, along with indirect costs, which includes lost productivity of both the survivors and the families involved. It is estimated that the indirect costs add as much as 35% to the total cost. Initial hospitalization cost is the largest percentage of direct costs, but hospital readmissions are calculated at 14%. Inpatient rehabilitation costs in 2009 were $5.7 billion, of which 27.9% were from stroke and TBI (AHA). In a study done at the University of Michigan, it is projected that the costs of stroke between 2005 and 2050 will reach $2.2 trillion. It is estimated that the heaviest burden for these costs will fall on the shoulders of the Hispanic and African American communities because, not only are they at higher risk, but also they tend to have a younger demographic stroke profile, which means a larger loss of productivity as younger people are taken out of the workforce.

Alternatives to family home care that might reduce the productivity cost to the family could include skilled nursing if the patient qualifies or assisted living for those who are more able. However, skilled-nursing facilities in California for example cost between $4,000 and $7,000 per month. (Some of that may be reimbursable by MediCal [in California] at the rate of between $125 and $550 per day if the patient qualifies.) The average length of stay nationwide is about 2.4 years. Assisted living, for those who are higher functioning, can range in cost from $1,500 to $6,000+ per month for the very spacious apartments and luxury settings. This might be appropriate for a mother or father, although there are instances of a husband and wife moving in together to ease the burden of care on the healthier of the two.

Home care aides may cost between $10 and $15 per hour based on level of service.

Yearly costs for each of these venues exceed the cost of care in the Stroke Recovery Center. SNF care can run as high as $48,000 to $84,000 per year while assisted living can run $18,000 to over $72,000 per year. Home care, which is the least expensive alternative, may run $20,400 to $21,200 for eight-hour coverage to allow the family member to be at work and, thereby, reduce some of the productivity losses. This is usually an out-of-pocket expense to the families.

On the other hand, the cost of care for a patient at the Stroke Recovery Center runs between $7,000 and $10,000 per year while reducing direct costs from readmissions and emergency room visits. The respite offered to families also acts to reduce the lost productivity numbers. Since the families are not asked to provide payment and the survivor receives therapy to aid in recovery, the benefits to the family, the benefits to the health-care system as a whole, and the benefits to productive society are calculable.

There is also a measurable benefit to be gained by the advocacy efforts of survivors and their families promoting stroke health and awareness. Who better to act as living examples of the issues involved in long-term care of stroke and TBI survivors than those who are living with the problems? Yet another benefit is the possible creation of services that may assist in the recovery in community settings and the gathering of peer groups to aid in sharing of resources and support for recovery. Cost and quality go hand in hand with the advocacy efforts, and even a small effort can have great results.

COMMUNITY ADVOCACY

While one may be inclined to turn inward after a stroke, turning outward is a better strategy to help energize recovery and to aid others in the same situation or, even better, help to prevent strokes. Education of others and the improvement of stroke treatment in your community are the goals of adding your voice to increase the volume and bring needed attention for more resources. Joining a stroke group is important to recovery. In that group, bring in the local hospital administrator, the local neurologists and internists, the local legislators, the state representatives, and even the federal legislators to talk with your group about the treatment of stroke and TBI survivors in your community.

Reach out to local schools, senior centers, and community groups to educate the population on stroke prevention and need for services. Promote research in stroke causation and treatment among the local universities and encourage participation. If there is no group in your area, start one. Raising awareness of stroke may result in the creation of stroke centers in hospitals and increase the quality of care throughout the nation so that patients may receive faster and better care wherever they may have their stroke or TBI.

ADVOCATING FOR A STROKE RECOVERY CENTER

This process presents a bigger challenge than community advocacy because of the cost of creating a center and the ongoing operational costs even though it is much less expensive than alternative forms of treatment. However, the potential outcome of creating a network of stroke recovery centers, each of which could create a hub for virtual presentation of services; covering the whole country with regional services to aid in long-term rehabilitation is well worth concerted efforts on the part of stroke survivors and their families.

To be an effective advocate, it is necessary to focus on the particular person/ organization that actually has the ability to implement the changes that you are advocating. Building awareness of the need for services and treatment supports the direct lobbying that can be done to the organizations that have the money and the motivation to initiate services but have not yet been educated to realize the potential for gain. To understand who those organizations are requires an understanding of how the health-care financing system works in the United States to determine who would best benefit from the creation and presentation of comprehensive services for stroke and TBI survivors and their families.

The major share of health-care dollars is currently spent on episodes of care. A physician sees a patient and bills insurance. A patient is in the hospital, and the hospital, the physician, the allied health professionals—the imaging, lab, and pharmacy—all bill the insurance company. The insurance company—either government Medicaid, Medicare, or TRICARE (the military) or private insurers like Blue Cross or Blue Shield—review the bill and pay a negotiate amount toward the total. As the patient, you may be responsible to pay for at least a portion of the remaining balance. Cost control over the health-care budget has been focused on negotiated rates along with denial of coverage. Denial of coverage or restriction of coverage have been draconian in terms of any type of long-term care or chronic care coverage, leaving needed therapies out of the reach of many patients and having the unintended consequence of moving care from less expensive modalities to more expensive modalities. For example, restrictions on in-home health-care reimbursement forces patients out of their homes into nursing homes that are reimbursed at a much higher level. In terms of stroke and TBI, lack of reimbursement for long-term rehabilitation leaves the patient at home with little hope for continued recovery.

However, there is a glimmer of hope in the Affordable Healthcare Act. While this reform is primarily focused on preserving the current system, there are some allowances for innovative funding systems and new projects that focus on longitudinal care, especially for chronic disease. This includes both ends of the care spectrum: prevention and long-term care. The current system offers no incentive for prevention or for long-term care in the private insurance realm because it is likely that the consumer will not be covered by the same employer-provided insurer for the long term. Why invest in prevention programs for a consumer who will switch to another insurer? The potential savings would accrue to the next or the next or even the next company down the line. Instead, the better business decision is to push the care down the line and let the government (Medicare) incur the heavy burden of end-of-life costs.

Under the new health plan, there are proposals to spread the responsibility of care over a longer period of the patient's life. Insurers will be responsible for preventive care, and hospitals and physicians working together will be responsible for the total care of the patient, including long-term care. Funding will shift from episodes of care to continuums of care, and care settings will include medical homes, community-based organizations, and home-based programs to assist in increasing the quality of care while reducing costs. There are a number of models that are currently funded as demonstration projects or under waivers from the federal government that offer opportunities to incorporate long-term rehabilitation treatment for stroke and TBI. A number of these will be detailed in the next section. Medicare will be leading the way in innovative payment mechanisms to incentivize providers to shift focus from disease management to patient-care management.

In the short-term, Medicare is fining hospitals for readmissions within thirty days for any reason. In the long term, Medicare will be reimbursing hospitals and physicians in bundled payments to treat a stroke or a TBI, and that payment will include allowances for aftercare. It is up to survivors and advocates for long-term care to make sure that organizations such as the Stroke Recovery Center are covered in such revisions of focus of the dollars. Making sure that the benefits shown by the research are communicated to hospitals, physicians, and politicians who can influence reimbursement scenarios can be accomplished with letter-writing campaigns, meetings with the stroke groups, and talking with individual providers.

Other avenues for reimbursement that currently is in place is the Medicare Advantage programs that currently exist as well as state-funded prepaid Medicaid programs. These programs provide a monthly payment to providers to give care to a patient. Usually contracted to a medical group, they are then responsible for the total care of the patient. The patient is likely to remain with the medical group for many years since he or she is elderly, disabled, or poor; therefore, the incentives to reduce costs over time are there for the medical group. Prevention, maintenance, and recovery all come into play in this scenario, and the focus shifts to quality of care and cost reduction as the patient is treated over time. Granted the patient may not be given all the care he or she wants—the physician may not authorize a prescription of that drug that was advertised on TV to do something wonderful—however, the patient will receive all the care that he or she needs. The emphasis is on health and wellness rather than on illness and disease. By understanding the benefit to chronic sufferers, introducing the addition of long-term rehabilitation to the treatment of stroke and TBI under this type of plan has the opportunity to revolutionize care.

MODELS OF CARE

Health-care reform shifts the focus from the episodes of care to make reasonable attempts to acknowledge and address access, inequalities, and delivery system reforms. The government is seeking innovation in payment structures and projects that will focus on comprehensive longitudinal care. Among the best practice models are increases in primary care payments that would also include a monthly payment, covered by insurance, in addition to a fee for service. This type of payment innovation would support what is referred to as patient-centered care. While not a new concept, patient-centered care is at the core of most of the models that are currently funded or being proposed. The model is focused on the primary care physician as the major component incorporating a team of providers to expand coverage of care. The patient-centered care model insures starts with access to care for the patient in terms of easy and accessible appointments, quick responses to issues, prescription information, and off-hours accessibility. The models ask that patients become engaged in their care and the decision-making process and provides for patient feedback. Care is coordinated with allied health professionals—specialists offering comprehensive, longitudinal care communicating electronically to track the patient among the team of providers. Among the models that incorporate this philosophy and offer opportunities to bring long-term treatment for stroke and TBI into the system are PACE (Project for All-inclusive Care for the Elderly), medical homes, safety-net clinic projects, and accountable care organizations.

The PACE program is a comprehensive care program for frail poor elderly designed to promote independent living and keep this at-risk population out of nursing homes and living in their own homes. To qualify, one must be over fifty-five years of age, nursing-home eligible, and be covered by Medicare with Medicaid as the secondary payer—MediMedi. This group may include a number of patients that would also be eligible for the Stroke Recovery Center but would also include patients with other diagnosis, including Alzheimer's. The program is center based with each facility housing medical, dental, physical therapy, recreational therapy, speech therapy, behavioral health services, and meals. Patients attend on an ambulatory basis, much the same manner as the Stroke Recovery Center patients. The care is coordinated through a care team of professionals who are responsible for primary, acute, and tertiary care, including hospitalizations, imaging, prescriptions, long-term care, meals-on-wheels, home care, and transportation to and from the center. Funding for the program is on a per-person-per-month basis with the patient having to qualify every six months to retain eligibility. Originally funded as a waiver program under Medicaid, PACE has achieved a success story that has warranted permanent waiver funding. Programs exist in a number of states, not all called PACE, but operating in the same manner. The National PACE Association, www.npaonline.org, works to provide a consistent voice for the facilities in Washington, DC. This program could value with an association with the Stroke Recovery Center using some shared space for the recreational programs, physical therapies, and exercise, along with shared meals. Additionally, the Stroke Recovery Center can serve as an upstream-development arm for future patients for PACE eligibility. This would make the conversion from the Stroke Recovery Center to the PACE program relatively seamless and very comfortable for the patients and the families involved. This model of concurrent programming is being tested in the current Stroke Recovery Center site.

Medical home is not just a building, house, or hospital but a team approach to providing health care. A medical home originates in a primary health-care setting that is family centered and compassionate. A partnership develops between the family and the primary health-care practitioner. Together they access all medical and nonmedical services needed by the child and family to achieve maximum potential. The medical home maintains a centralized, comprehensive record of all health-related services to promote continuity of care. In other words, patient-centered care works from the primary care provider's office and incorporates the comprehensive team by electronically tying them together to provide primary, acute, chronic, and preventive care. Reimbursement models are being tested; however, the original model was tested and is used in Denmark, and the method of reimbursement they have successfully used is to combine a monthly fee with a fee for specific professional services. The monthly fees would support programs like the Stroke Recovery Center that could act as a provider for a number of patients being treated under the medical home model and be a functional part of the care team connected electronically and participating in the coordination of care.

Safety-net clinics deliver a range of primary and specialty care to medically underserved and uninsured people regardless of their ability to pay. They have been indispensible in improving care to this at-risk population and have offered innovative care delivery methods, such as chronic disease management, service integration, and telemedicine—all designed to integrate care and increase quality. A key characteristic of a number of innovative care models is the colocation of a range of health-care services and community services in one site. Generally, there are two levels of colocation: consolidation of various health-care services including primary care, dental, behavioral health, and social work; and consolidation of health-care services with other community services including school, community center, and retail. By providing one-stop care, there are economies of scale to both the patient and the provider and provision of a more holistic approach of focusing on the entire person and lending of the ability to coordinate care, particularly in the case of multiple diagnosis (comorbidities). Several of these safety-net clinic community centers are being tested and would lend themselves to a stroke recovery center component. Funding for these clinics has typically been on a cost basis, and provision of rehabilitation services to the poor and underserved might offer additional opportunities for revenue along with increasing the quality of care.

Accountable care organizations are written into the Affordable Healthcare Act to provide longitudinal services to patient-integrating care from primary to long-term care. While still under development, the concept offers an opportunity for providers to develop the areas of lower profitability—the community-based services—as a part of an integrated delivery system that includes physicians, hospitals, ancillary providers, and long-term care options. Payment and oversight could be instituted at the management level of the ACO itself to ensure quality standards and compliance to evidence-based practice parameters.

Services for stroke and TBI survivors should to be based on community need. However, as noted earlier, the survival rate for strokes strongly suggests that the three million people who are estimated to be living with stroke is not exaggerated. Among these innovative programs, there needs to be an awareness of the benefit of adding stroke recovery to the care mix and incorporating a program not currently in the continuum of care.

SOCIAL NETWORKING AND ADVOCACY

The Internet offers a platform for advocacy. Building a network of survivors all working toward recovery, having local groups banded together throughout the country, and demonstrating the thriving of survivors as they respond to rehabilitation, not only makes a convincing argument, but helps the recovery of the patients and their families. The use of YouTube and Facebook to build networks is an excellent start. The connection to and the involvement in the virtual clinic at www.strokerecoverycenter.org is an important part of networking. While the services are limited online, as time goes on, the ability to interface with other survivors across the country and the world will build a far-reaching network, identifying needs and available help. As stroke recovery centers develop and more regions are able to join the conversation, the critical mass will develop to make this population a viable force for change.

AFTERWORD

For more information please visit our website, www.strokerecoverycenter.org, or give us a call at 760-323-7676. We have been delivering services to survivors for over thirty years and hope to continue for at least another thirty years and are appalled that there are so few options open to this population. By working together, we can make a difference.

NOTES

1. Stroke Statistics, TheUniversityHospital.com.

2. Ibid.

3. Ibid.

4. HARC (Health Assessment Resource Center), <u>Community Health Monitor 2007.</u>

5. Kaiser-Commonwealth Study, 2002.

6. HARC, Community..

7. Eric W. Nawar, R. W. Nisha, and Jianmin Xu, *National Hospital Ambulatory Medical Care Survey: 2005 Emergency Department Summary,* CDC Advance Data # 386, June 29, 2007.

8. S. R. Machlin, "Expenses for a Hospital Emergency Visit, 2003." Agency for Healthcare Research and Quality Statistical Brief #111, January 2006.

9. Archstone Foundation, *California Blueprint for Fall Prevention* (white paper presented at the Archstone Foundation Conference, February 2003).

10. HARC, Community.

11. Archstone, *California.*

REFERENCES

Chapter I: What You Need to Know About Strokes and TBI

What Happens When Someone Has a Stroke or TBI?

1. Jean-Dominique Bauby, *The Diving Bell and the Butterfly* (New York: Alfred A. Knopf, 1997), 4.

2. Jill Bolte Taylor, *My Stroke of Insight* (New York: the Penguin Group, 2006), 78–79.

3. Doris W. Braley, *Stroke: The Road Back* (Portland: Harbor House West, 1994), 8–9.

4. Alison Bonds Shapiro, *Healing into Possibility* (Tiberon, CA: HJ Kramer, 2009), 8.

How Do People React to Having a Stroke?

5. Jill Bolte Taylor, *My Stroke of Insight* (New York: the Penguin Group, 2006), 78.

6. Jean-Dominique Bauby, *The Diving Bell and the Butterfly* (New York: Alfred A. Knopf, 1997), 110.

7. Doris W. Braley, *Stroke: The Road Back* (Portland: Harbor House West, 1994), 13.

8. Julia Fox Garrison, *Don't Leave Me This Way* (New York: Harper, 2007), 52.

9. Ibid., 48.

Acute Rehabilitation

One Other Issue

10. Alison Bonds Shapiro, *Healing into Possibility* (Tiberon, CA: HJ Kramer, 2009).

11. Jill Bolte Taylor, *My Stroke of Insight* (New York: the Penguin Group, 2006).

12. Ibid.

Where Do You Get Help?

13. Jean-Dominique Bauby, *The Diving Bell and the Butterfly* (New York: Alfred A. Knopf, 1997), 40.

14. Julia Fox Garrison, *Don't Leave Me This Way* (New York: Harper, 2007), 214.

15. Alison Bonds Shapiro, *Healing into Possibility* (Tiberon, CA: HJ Kramer, 2009), 8.

16. Doris W. Braley, *Stroke: The Road Back* (Portland: Harbor House West, 1994), 32.

Communities and Organizations

17. Jill Bolte Taylor, *My Stroke of Insight* (New York: the Penguin Group, 2006), 82.

18. Julia Fox Garrison, *Don't Leave Me This Way* (New York: Harper, 2007).

19. Ibid.

Caregivers and Patients

20. Jill Bolte Taylor, *My Stroke of Insight* (New York: the Penguin Group, 2006).

21. Alison Bonds Shapiro, *Healing into Possibility* (Tiberon, CA: HJ Kramer, 2009), 206–207.

22. Jill Bolte Taylor, *My Stroke of Insight* (New York: the Penguin Group, 2006).

23. Julia Fox Garrison, *Don't Leave Me This Way* (New York: Harper, 2007), 164.

24. Ibid.

25. Alison Bonds Shapiro, *Healing into Possibility* (Tiberon, CA: HJ Kramer, 2009), 209.

Success Factors

26. Jill Bolte Taylor, *My Stroke of Insight* (New York: the Penguin Group, 2006), 78.

27. Norman Doidge, *The Brain that Changes Itself* (New York: the Penguin Group, 2007), 148–149.

Alternative Therapies

28. Julia Fox Garrison, *Don't Leave Me This Way* (New York: Harper, 2007), 211.

APPENDIXES

Research 2007

Research 2008

Research 2009

Sample Menu

Sample Activities

Website Home Page

Sample Statistical Report

STROKE RECOVERY CENTER

Organizational Health Initiative Project

December 2007

Prepared March 2008

Funding provided by the Desert Healthcare District

CONTENTS

1. Executive Summary 105

2. Organizational Health Initiative Project 109
    a. Introduction 109
    b. Philosophy 109
    c. Treatment Options 110

3. Research Design and Parameters 111

4. Results 114
    a. Age and Sex of Clients 114
    b. Body Mass Index 116
    c. Type of Stroke and Frequency Measurement 117
    d. Comorbidities and Prescription Drug Usage 118
    e. Number of Persons in the Household 119
    f. Transportation 120
    g. Ambulation 121
    h. Orthotics 122
    i. Emergency Room Visits 123
    j. Falls 124

5. Conclusions 126

6. Sources 128

EXECUTIVE SUMMARY

Organizational Health Initiative Project

The Organizational Health Initiative Project (OHIP) that the Stroke Recovery Center (SRC) is undertaking is designed to position the services of the center as a valued component in the continuing care (the continuum of care) for stroke victims. The OHIP methodology is to gather data of critical factors for chronic stroke treatment from the existing patient base and compare such data to stroke victims who have limited access to rehabilitative programs. The project objective is to develop a client data tracking system that will be used to prove the economic and social value of long-term stroke rehabilitation. The hypothesis to be tested is that stroke victims who use the Stroke Recovery Center are less of a financial burden on the health and social service budgets than those who do not access Stroke Recovery Center services. The Stroke Recovery Center, as the best practice model for continuing care for stroke survivors, requires eligibility for predictable and sustainable funding from government, private insurance, and/or medical group providers to be replicated in other locations.

Research Design and Parameters

We have collected and tabulated data from 95 clients who, as of February 1, 2008, were Stroke Recovery Center users, having been there 3+ months and attended at least three times per month or more. Measurement of the utilization data offers the most compelling evidence of recovery.

The initial baseline data was analyzed using the criteria of length of attendance (LOS) at the Stroke Recovery Center. While 37% of the group have been attending less than a full year, 47% have attended between 1 and 5 years. The heaviest concentration of clients tends to be in the 2- and 3-year area that suggests that once the client makes the commitment to stay with the program beyond the first year, they tend to stay with us for 1 to 2 years. The drop-off occurs after 4 years. This may be due to a number of factors, not the least of which is the aging issue. With the median LOS at 2 years, data points in the categories listed below were compared to determine if there were differences in the early users as compared to those who have been at the center for 2+ years.

Results

The data findings were addressed in the following categories:

Age and sex of clients. The average age of clients attending is 68 years of age with a median of 70 years of age. The standard deviation is 12 years, which means that using a normal distribution, 68% of the client base is between 58 and 80 years of age. As expected, the group attending 2+ years has a median age 3 years older than the group who has attended less than 2 years. The client base is 58% males and 42% females. Males tend to stay with the program longer, becoming 65% in the group attending 2+ years.

Body mass index (BMI). BMI is an indicator of the amount of body fat by measuring the ratio between one's height and weight adjusted by age and sex. The body fat index is considered to be related to the risk of disease and death. The average BMI of clients is slightly higher than the national norm of 18.5–24.9, suggesting that the Stroke Recovery Center is not doing enough in weight control and nutrition since it appears BMI is increasing with the length of time spent at the center. Since most of the group is at high risk with additional factors, the importance of the nutritional program is evident.

Comorbidities and prescription drugs. The most prevalent comorbidity is hypertension with 58% of the client population reporting it. The average number of drugs taken by the client population is 4.5 per day. While there appears to be no correlation to the length of attendance at the center, this is an indicator that needs to be analyzed in more detail to determine if drug interventions should become part of the program that is presented. An increase of one drug per day is movement in a negative direction as the time passes, and while it may be age related, it warrants further tracking to see if it holds up over time.

Number of persons in household. Data shows 79% of clients live with another person in the household but does indicate that a higher percentage of clients who continue to come to the center live alone—24% compared to 21%.

Ambulation. Differences in ambulation and ambulation aids show a movement from walkers to canes from those who spend a longer time at the center than from those that are in the first two years.

Orthotics. Orthotics are typically used to assist in drop foot, which increases difficulty in walking. The decrease in orthotic usage may be related to the ambulation-assistance devices cited above.

Transportation. There are three major types of transportation modes that the clients use to access the Stroke Recovery Center: the SunDial bus, a home pickup and delivery for handicapped persons that services the Coachella Valley; family and/or caregivers, which include the specialty vans that bring clients from assisted living homes or serve as taxis to the handicapped; and there are a number of clients who are able to drive themselves. With the group who has attended less than 2 years, there is a heavy reliance on family and/or caregivers—61%. Once the clients have been at the center longer, there is a shift toward the SunDial bus with 27% of longer-term users riding the bus as well as those who drive themselves—31%. At the same time, reliance on family and/or caregivers goes down to 42%. This may indicate an increased self-reliance and independence that is attributable to those clients who remain at the Stroke Recovery Center.

Emergency room visits. In the last year, 2007, 32% of the client population made at least one trip to an emergency room for service. Of that number, 13% were clients who have been at the center more than 2 years while 87% were clients who have been at the center less than 2 years. Using the rate and median cost, the annual cost for ER visits would be $9,344 per 100 persons. The client population at the Stroke Recovery Center would be $8,098 per 100 persons for those who have attended less than 2 years and $1,226 per 100 persons for those who have a longer length of attendance. This is a significant difference and major long-term care cost saving.

Falls. As much as 30% of the client population suffered from a fall in the past year, 2007. Estimated medical costs for a senior-fall-related hospitalization in California is $30,000. The group of clients that have been with the center less than 2 years suffered falls at nearly double the rate of those who have been at the center longer.

Conclusions

Benefits to the clients who participate in the programs at the Stroke Recovery Center for more than 2 years indicate growing recovery of independence and self-reliance. While results are not linear, they strongly suggest that, even though the population ages, they are maintaining a great level of recovery than from those who attend less than 2 years.

This program offers savings to the long-term care of stroke survivors by offering a nonclinical and inexpensive alternative, reducing higher costs of emergency room visits, hospitalizations, and physician fees. As a model for care, this type of program should become fundable and, thereby, replicable.

ORGANIZATIONAL HEALTH INITIATIVE PROJECT

Introduction

The Organizational Health Initiative Project (OHIP) of the Stroke Recovery Center (SRC) is designed to position the services of the center as a valued component in the continuing care (the continuum of care) for stroke victims. The OHIP methodology is to gather data of critical factors for chronic stroke treatment from our existing patient base and compare such data to stroke victims who do not access the rehabilitative programs. The project objective is to develop a client data tracking system that will be used to prove the economic and social value of long-term stroke rehabilitation as practiced at the Stroke Recovery Center. The hypothesis to be tested is that stroke victims who use the Stroke Recovery Center are less of a financial burden on the health and social service budgets than those who do not access Stroke Recovery Center services.

The Stroke Recovery Center is a nonclinical, inexpensive combination of programs that offers long-term rehabilitation to the survivors of stroke along with support for their families, caregivers, and loved ones. The center is unique in that it provides services at no cost to the stroke survivor or his/her family once health benefits have been depleted. Having an operational budget of approximately $650,000 (the center owns its own building), the center relies exclusively on fund-raising events, foundation and family donations, and revenues from its on-site thrift shop to fund the services it provides to over 225 clients per year, five days per week, on an ambulatory basis. As mentioned before, the Organizational Health Initiative Project is designed to position the Stroke Recovery Center as a valued part of the continuum of care and, as a best practice model, become eligible for predictable and sustainable funding from government, private insurance, and/or medical group providers.

Philosophy

The Stroke Recovery Center focuses on treatment of the whole person, offering a safe environment with respect given each client and his/her family and loved ones. Staff works with each client, recognizing the humanity within each client regardless of the severity of their impairment. The center works with the imagination, the humor, the anger, the depression, and the sexuality of each client along with the specific physical, cognitive, and communication disorder that may exist. The philosophy of the center focuses on treatment of the mind, the body, and the spirit, challenging the physical, the aesthetic, and the mental capabilities of each of our clients combined with social interaction and just plain fun.

Treatment Options

The center offers exercise therapy focusing on balance and strengthening of the weak side with both individual and group treatments. Speech therapy is offered on an individual and group basis along with computer-assisted communication therapy using both individual programs and computers designed to assist communication. Recreational therapists offer a schedule of activities to fill the day. These programs vary from rap sessions on current events, group sessions on dealing with recovery issues, improvisational theater, arts and crafts, computer usage and Wii, to entertainment and bingo. The programs are designed to promote interaction and peer support development along with cognitive improvement.

Programs are offered Monday through Friday from 9:30 AM to 2:00 PM with a hot lunch served at 12:30 PM daily if the clients wish to partake. Clients are allowed to attend programs of their choosing. Exercise therapy requires a physician's release.

RESEARCH DESIGN AND PARAMETERS

Design

We have collected and tabulated data from 95 clients who, as of February 1, 2008, were Stroke Recovery Center users, having been here 3+ months and attend at least 3 times per month or more. This group of clients is representative of the client base as a whole and has been subject to both initial questioning regarding the utilization issues and, in most cases, one follow-up that we have used to form the baseline data for the year-end 2007 and will be the data for comparison going forward.

We had also instituted a psychosocial-scale instrument that we received from the National Stroke Association and have been adding that to the client's medical record. However, after review of the initial data, we have abandoned that instrument, which, although interesting, deals primarily with the issue of depression. As we know, depression is very common among stroke survivors, and it is our contention that we have a very positive effect on poststroke depression along with our positive value to the families and caregivers in dealing with the effects of stroke. In administering this scale to our population, we found results become positive in the first 3 months after their evaluations. We feel that it is equally important to deal with this aspect of stroke recovery as it is to deal with the physical and speech problems, and it is an important part of our therapy.

However, what makes the Stroke Recovery Center unique is that we combine treatments working on the emotional and spiritual elements of the survivor's humanity with physical and cognitive and communication issues.

It is that uniqueness that we measured to derive quantitative outcomes. Because of the initial results of the data, we decided that the measurement of the utilization data offers the most compelling and supportable evidence of recovery. The measurements we achieved from the scales, we believe, are reflected in the utilization data reported. In other words, the scale data improvements (i.e., the easing of depression) help to enable the achievements we have documented in the utilization data. For that reason, we have decided to go forward with the collection and analysis of the utilization data as opposed to collecting the scale data.

Parameters

The baseline data is analyzed using the criteria of length of attendance (LOS) to the center. This parameter is chosen to determine if clients show improvement over time spent at the center and partaking in the programs. To support this as the supporting factor to recovery, the data is also analyzed and adjusted for age variations, comorbidities, type of stroke, and length of time since the last stroke. The initial group varies in the LOS from the 3 months threshold to 13 years.

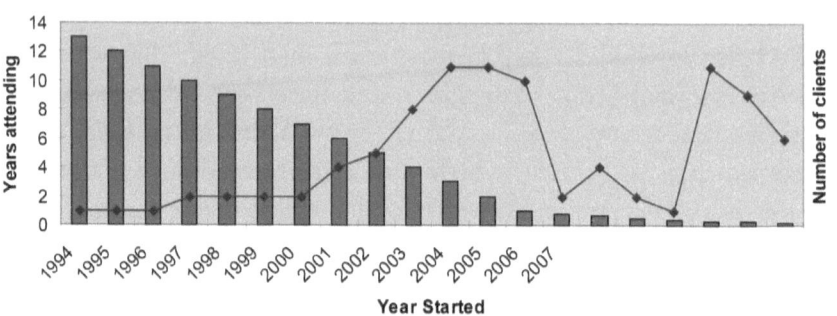

The 95 clients in the baseline group have an average (mean) length of attendance at the center of 2.79 years with a standard deviation of 2.99. The mean is the number of years and/or months divided by the number of clients, and the standard deviation measures the spread in the data set. This means that the spread is so great that the mean is highly influenced by the outliers—we show 8 clients at 9+ years—that a more meaningful measurement is the median 2.0 years. The median is the middle of the data set and has an equal number of data points above and below the median value.

Therefore, going forward with our analysis, we will use the median number of 2 years attendance and compare the greater than (>) 2 year attendees to the less than (<) 2 year attendees.

While 37% of the group have been attending less than a full year, 47% have attended between 1 and 5 years. The heaviest concentration of clients tends to be in the 2 and 3 year area, which suggests that once the client makes the commitment to stay with the program beyond the first year, they tend to stay with us for 1 to 2 more years. The drop-off occurs after 4 years. This may be due to a number of factors, not the least of which is the aging issue; however, this is an element that needs further study and documentation.

We looked at the following data based on the client's length of attendance:

- Age and sex
- Body mass index
- Numbers in household
- Transportation
- Comorbidities and drug usage
- Ambulation
- Orthotic usage
- ER visits
- Number of falls

RESULTS

Age and Sex of Clients

The average age of clients attending is 68 years of age with a median of 70 years of age. The standard deviation is 12 years, which means that using a normal distribution, 68% of the client base is between 58 and 80 years of age. On the other hand, it also indicates that 16% are either over 80 years of age or less than 58 years of age. This is indicative of the wide range of ages that can and are affected by stroke; however, stroke risk increases with age. For each decade after the age of 55, the risk of stroke doubles.[1] Since only 28% of stroke victims are less than 65 years of age nationally, our overall population at the Stroke Recovery Center is slightly younger than the national norms for stroke would suggest.

The group that has attended less than 2 years has a mean age of 67 with the median 68 years of age. As would be expected, the group that has attended longer than 2 years is older with an average (mean) age of 70.6 years of age and a median age of 71 years. Using standard deviations of the two groups, the age spread of the less-than-2-year group is 54 years of age to 80 years of age while the age spread of those who have attended over 2 years is 60 years of age to 80 years of age. Overlaying this to the results suggests that improvements that are made are not age dependent.

The sex of the client base is more closely aligned with national norms. The client base is 58% males and 42% females. Women account for 43% of strokes each year according to national data. However, they also account for 61% of the deaths.[2]

Sex of clients LOS under 2 Years

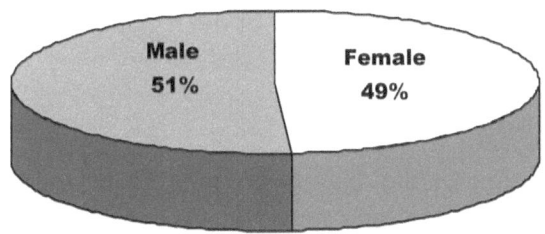

Among the clients who have attended less than 2 years, the numbers are almost equal: 49% women and 51% men. However, for those who have been here longer than 2 years, the percentage changes to 35% women and 65% men.

Sex of clients LOS over 2 Years

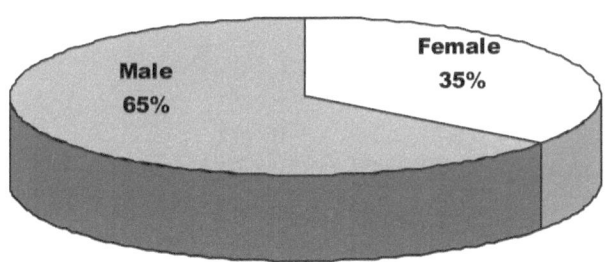

The incident rate for stroke varies by ethnicity. In Caucasian males, the rate is 62.8 per 100,000; for females, the rate is 59 per 100,000. For Afro American males, the rate is 93 per 100,000 and 79 per 100,000 for females. Prevalence for those over 20 years of age for non-Hispanic white men is

2.2%, women is 1.5%; for non-Hispanic black men is 2.5%, women is 3.2%; and for Mexican American men is 2.3%, women is 1.3%.[3] As the number of clients in the database grows, the center should be able to track the ethnicity of the client base as it compares to national norms and also as it compares to the general population of the region.

Body Mass Index

BMI is an indicator of the amount of body fat by measuring the ratio between one's height and weight adjusted by age and sex. The body fat index is considered to be related to the risk of disease and death. A limitation that affects the Stroke Recovery Center's population is the risk of underestimating the body fat in older persons or those who have lost muscle mass that will occur with stroke. However, the norms are the following: normal is 18.5–24.9, overweight is 25.0–29.9, and obese is 30+. Other risk factors that add to the risk are hypertension, high cholesterol, inactivity, and smoking.

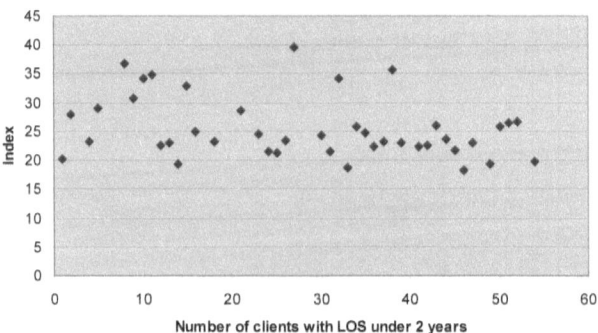

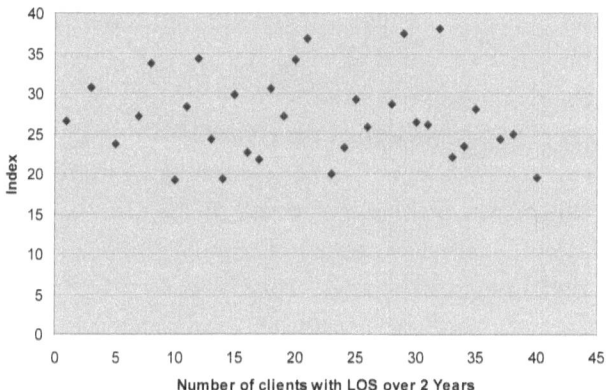

The average (mean) BMI for those who have been attending less than 2 years is 25.5, slightly overweight. The median is 23.6, normal. For those who have attended longer, the BMI increases to average (mean) 27, overweight. The median for this group is 26.5, also overweight. Assuming a degree of undercounting due to loss of muscle mass, this suggests the Stroke Recovery Center is not doing enough in weight control and nutrition since it appears BMI is increasing with the length of time spent at the center. Since most of the group is at high risk with the additional factors, the importance of our nutrition and exercise programs is a high level of concern going forward.

According to data collected by HARC (Health Assessment Resource Center), 39.1% of seniors in the Eastern Coachella Valley are overweight and 15.7% are obese.[4] The center's population tends to be more heavily obese (38%) as well as overweight (47%).

Type of Stroke and Frequency Measurement

Of the two types of stroke, the ischemic is more prevalent than the hemorrhagic. There are a total of 20 hemorrhagic strokes in the research group—11 in the group who have attended over 2 years and 9 in the group that have attended less than 2 years. Since the difference in the groups is small, the influence of the type of stroke over the results is probably limited.

Also of interest is the amount of time since the last stroke. One would suspect that the passage of time would have a great influence on recovery. However, looking at the comparison between our two groups, those that have been at the center for over 2 years are 6.4 years past their last strokes with a median of 5 years and a standard deviation of 4.4 years. On the other hand, those who have been at the center less than 2 years are 3.2 years past their last stroke with a median of 1 year and standard deviation of 5.7 years. What this means is there is a spread in the first group of 2–10 years poststroke and 0–9 years poststroke in the later group. In other words, the influence of the time spent at the Stroke Recovery Center appears to be greater than the time since the last stroke. It is interesting to note that those who are just starting at the center may be as long as 9 years poststroke, and we are still able to demonstrate positive results.

Comorbidities and Prescription Drug Usage

The most prevalent comorbidity is hypertension with 58% of the client population reporting it. Heart problems are the second most reported with 47% of the population. Chronic pain is reported by 21%, and severe headaches are reported by 19%. Arthritis is reported by 38% of the population, which may also be related to the age of the group. There is an array of other major diseases, such as Parkinson's, cancer, HIV, prostate cancer, osteoporosis, and seizures. Quantifying comorbidities by the major groups of heart, cancer, diabetes, and AIDS, the data is the same in both groups of those who have attended greater or lesser than 2 years. The mean is 0.57 with a standard deviation of 0.66, which means that clients tend to suffer from comorbidities at a consistent rate.

In a study done by Kaiser, they found that patients suffering from 3+ chronic health problems, 75% of the patients took 7 or more prescription drugs per day.[5] The average usage by all seniors is less.

None: 18%

1–2:   36%

3–4:   25%

5+:   21%

The average (mean) number of drugs taken by the client population is 4.5 per day with a median of 5 and standard deviation of 3, which indicated a number of significant outliers that are attributable to comorbidities. Because of this, the median of 5 is the more appropriate number to use. In looking at the median in the less-than-2-year group compared to the more-than-2-year group, the number increases from 4 to 5. While there appears to be no correlation to the length of attendance at the center, this is an indicator that needs to be analyzed in more detail to determine if drug interventions should become part of the program that is presented. An increase of 1 drug per day is movement in a negative direction as the time passes, and while it may be age related, since there is virtually no difference in comorbidities, it warrants further tracking.

Number of Persons in the Household

Only 21% of the client base lives alone. This is lower than the 27.1% Eastern Coachella Valley residents reported to HARC (Health Assessment Resource Center).[6] Of those, a higher percentage have been at the center over 2 years, 24% as compared to 18% who are in their first 2 years. While this is not a large number difference, it may be said that those who are more independent do tend to stay at the center longer.

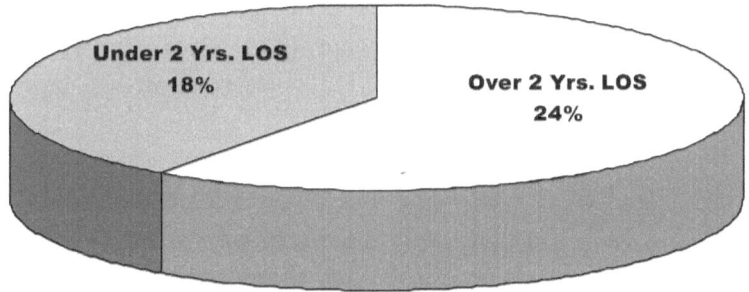

Clients who live alone

Transportation

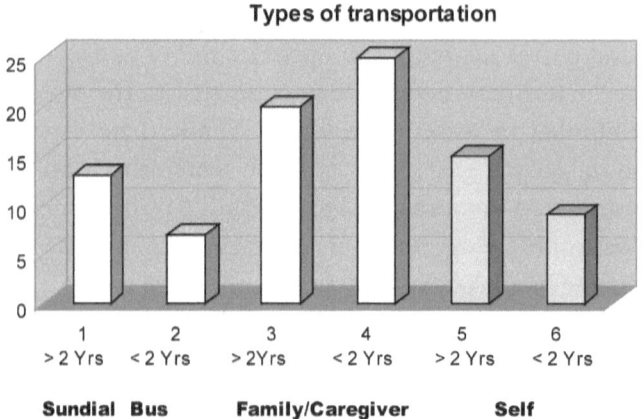

There are three major types of transportation modes that the clients use to access the Stroke Recovery Center: the SunDial bus, which is a home pickup and delivery for handicapped persons that services the Coachella Valley; family and/or caregivers, which include the specialty vans than bring clients from assisted living homes or serve as taxis to the handicapped; and there are a number of clients who are able to drive themselves.

With the group who has attended less than 2 years, there is a heavy reliance on family and/or caregivers—61%. Only 17% are using the SunDial bus, and another 22% are able to drive themselves. The SunDial bus requires a degree of self-reliance—pickups are scheduled within a forty-minute window, and clients must be outside waiting for the driver, which means that they usually can get in and out of their homes unassisted. It also costs $1 each way for Palm Springs residents and $2 each way for nonresidents.

Once the clients have been at the center longer, there is a shift toward the SunDial bus with 27% of longer-term users riding the bus as well as those who drive themselves—31%. At the same time, reliance on family and/or caregivers goes down to 42%. This may indicate that there is an increased self-reliance and independence that is attributable to those clients who remain at the Stroke Recovery Center.

Ambulation

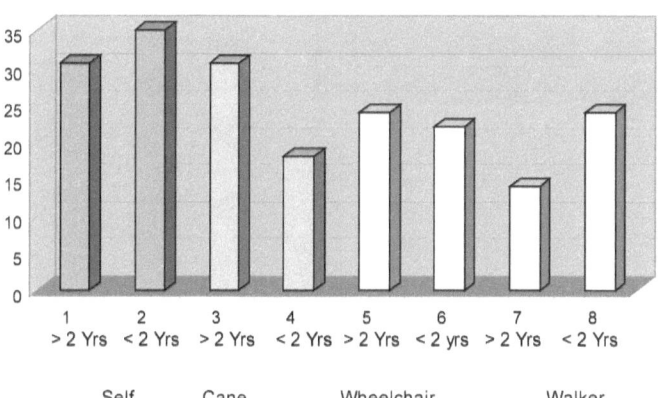

Differences in ambulation and ambulation aids show less difference between those who spend a longer time at the center than from those that are in the first 2 years. The two biggest differences are in the use of canes that increases as time goes on (18%–30.5%) and walker use (24%–14%) that seems to lessen with time. Wheelchair usage and self-ambulation seem to remain somewhat static, 22%–25% and 35%–39% respectively. This may be a factor of the aging process more than a result of the continued exercise therapy.

Orthotics

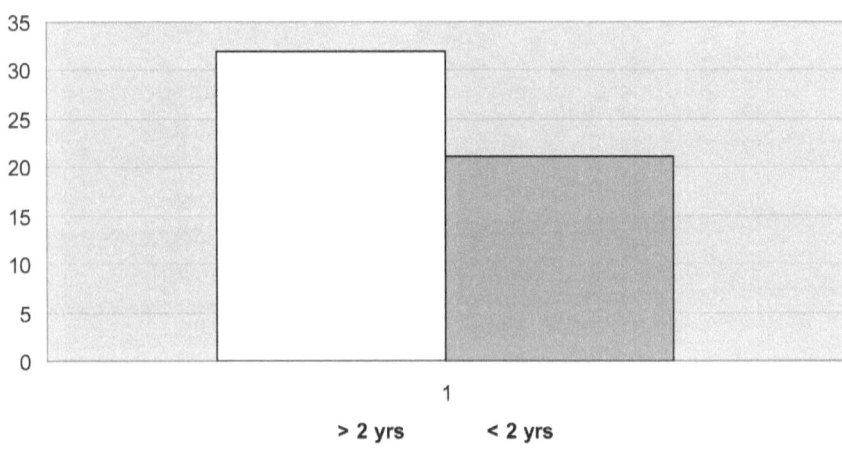

Of the clients that have been at the center more than 2 years, 21% wear orthotics on their leg and/or arm. Of those who have been at the center less than 2 years, 32% wear orthotics on their leg and/or arm. Orthotics are typically used to assist in drop foot, which increase difficulty in walking. The decrease in orthotic usage may be related to the ambulation-assistance devices cited above and should be tracked over time.

Orthotics are typically paid for, at least in part, by Medicare and vary according to the level of sophistication of the appliance. There are numerous electronically assisted aids to mobility that are promoted to the stroke community that tend to be expensive and out of the reach of most of our client base. However, there are at least two of our clients who have purchased an electronically assisted muscle stimulator that is strapped below the knee and assists with drop foot. The unit costs $5,000, and the results have been mixed from good outcomes to negative outcomes. The negative outcome has been that the devise overtires the user rather than assists him/her. There is not yet any indication of the device improving the neurological function.

Emergency Room Visits

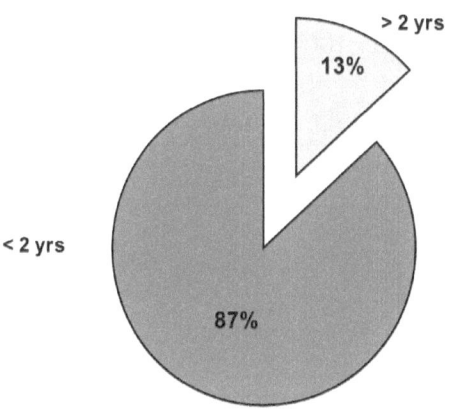

ER Visits in the last year

In the last year, 2007, 32% of the client population made at least one trip to an emergency room for service. Of that number, 13% were clients who have been at the center more than 2 years while 87% were clients who have been at the center less than 2 years. This is a significant difference and major long-term care cost saving that should be tracked over time to see if it will continue.

In the latest reported year of 2005, ER visits were recorded at 39.6 per 100 persons, according to data from the US Department of Health and Human Services.[7] Incidents for Hispanics are higher—40.0 per 100—as compared to 39.5 for non-Hispanics. Overall, women have a higher rate—41.8 per 100—as opposed to men—37.4 per 100—with those over 75 years of age significantly higher at 59.4 and 59.8 respectively. Whites are at 36.8 per 100, blacks at 69.0 per 100, Asians at 17.2 per 100, and Native Americans at 28.0 per 100. While these data are age related and insurance coverage related as well as related by type of presenting problem, the number of visits in one year noted by our client population is 30, which converts to 31.25 per 100—lower than the national norm. Considering the advanced age of the population, this is considerably lower even with the group that has been attending less than 2 years.

Cost for ER visits according to a study by the Agency for Healthcare Research and Quality show that in 2003, the average cost was $560.[8] The range of cost was from $42 to $1,246; therefore, the median cost of $299 is a more useful number to use. The cost is higher for those between the ages of 45 and 64—$832. Using the rate and median cost, the annual cost for ER visits would be $9,344 per 100 persons. The client population at the Stroke Recovery Center would be $8,098 per 100 persons for those who have attended less than 2 years and $1,226 per 100 persons for those who have a longer length of attendance.

Falls

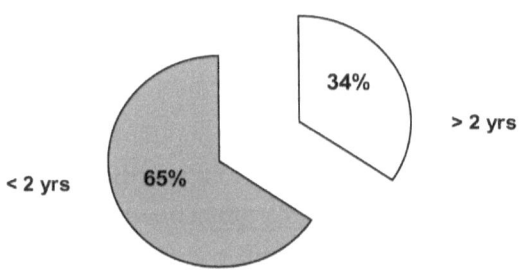

As much as 30% of the client population suffered from a fall in the past year, 2007.[9] The group of clients that have been with the center less than 2 years suffered falls at nearly double the rate of those who have been at the center longer. In percentages, 34% of the clients who fell have been at the center longer than 2 years while 65% of those who fell have been at the center less than 2 years. This number will have to be tracked over time and, if it proves out, will be a significant benefit to long-term, chronic care management.

It is estimated that 30% of older Californians fall each year, although HARC (Health Assessment Resource Center) reported only 12% of residents of the eastern Coachella Valley had fallen in the prior 3-month period.[10] In a white paper presented to the CA Blueprint for Fall Prevention Conference sponsored by the Archstone Foundation, the risk factors for falling include leg weakness, gait and balance problems, previous falls, general functional impairment, visual deficits, cognitive impairments, depression, taking psychoactive medications, and taking more than 4 different prescription medications. Estimated medical costs for a senior-fall-related hospitalization in California is $30,000.[11]

In 2007, the client population of the Stroke Recovery Center was consistent with this national 30% number, recording falls by 30.2% of the group. Breaking the numbers down to those who have been in attendance longer than 2 years, the percentage of falls goes down to 10.4% while the group who has attended less than 2 years records falls at the rate of 19.8%. With the client population fulfilling at least one and usually more of the risk factors, the results are even more impressive.

CONCLUSIONS

Analysis of the data strongly suggests the benefits to stroke survivors of participating long term in a program designed to support continued recovery. Support for this contention is indicated specifically in the results of the number of persons in the household and the transportation data. Although the differences are small, the data is suggesting that those who have been with the program longer are able to live alone more so than those who are early to the program. Movement of the numbers of clients to more independent means of transportation, both buses and driving, suggests a higher level of independence for those who have been coming to the center longer.

The value of the center as a functional intervention in the continuum of care for stroke survivors may be supported by the data for ambulation, orthotics, emergency room visits, and falls. Ambulation toward single canes as opposed to walkers suggests a higher level of confidence and independence and supports the fall data that is very significant in comparison to the data for falls in the elderly population as a whole. These numbers translate to dollar savings for the health-care system and dovetail with the emergency room visit reductions we see in the group going forward in the program. Falls cost the system money, not only in ER visits, but in caregiver costs, SNF costs, rehab costs, hospital stays, physician costs, DME, and other orthotics. The orthotic use in the Stroke Recovery Center group follows the same trend as the other data, indicating the importance of continued participation in the program.

On the other hand, it is important to note that a correlation between the amount of time spent at Stroke Recovery Center and improvement in the numbers is not statistically significant. In other words, we are unable to say either that the longer one stays with the program, the better he/she will be, nor are we able to say that the program causes less falls, lowers emergency room usage, etc. However, we are also unable to correlate these improvements to age, type of stroke, passage of time since the stroke, or comorbidities. By eliminating linear regression of the possible causative elements, we are left with the common factor variation that is most significant being the time spent in the program with one's peer group as having the greatest influence on recovery as measured by these parameters. Taking the advancing age of the individual as he/she continues to attend the center, the results we have posted become even more significant. It is possible to posit that, while unable to support a linear relationship, we are able to demonstrate recovery and maintenance of improvement as the client continues to age. This outcome is of high value to the elderly population.

It is our contention that over the period of the next few years, the data will strengthen the position and support the efficacy of this type of nonclinical, inexpensive intervention to stroke victims throughout the country as a fundable component of stroke long term.

For information contact

Beverly Greer
CEO
Stroke Recovery Center
(760) 323-7676
bgreer@strokerecoverycenter.org

SOURCES

California Blueprint for Fall Prevention, Archstone Foundation Conference White Paper, February 2003.

Nawar, Eric W., R. W. Nisha, and Jianmin Xu. *National Hospital Ambulatory Medical Care Survey: 2005 Emergency Department Summary.* CDC Advance Data # 386, June 29, 2007.

Health Assessment Resource Center (HARC). Community Health Monitor. 2007.

Kaiser-Commonwealth Study, 2002.

S. R. Machlin. "Expenses for a Hospital Emergency Visit, 2003." Agency for Healthcare Research and Quality Statistical Brief #111, January 2006.

Stroke Statistics. TheUniversityHospital.com.

STROKE RECOVERY CENTER

Update to
Organizational Health Initiative Project

December 2008

Prepared May 2009

CONTENTS

1. Executive Summary 131
2. Organizational Health Initiative Project 135
3. Research Design and Parameters 136
4. Results 138
   a. Age and Sex of Clients... 138
   b. Prescription Drug Usage.. 140
   c. Transportation 140
   d. Ambulation 142
   e. Orthotics.. 143
   f. Emergency Room Visits 144
   g. Falls 145
5. Conclusions 146

EXECUTIVE SUMMARY

Organizational Health Initiative Project

The Organizational Health Initiative Project (OHIP) is now in its second year of data gathering and analysis. The OHIP methodology is to gather data regarding outcomes of treatment for chronic stroke suffers from the existing patient base and compare such data to stroke victims who are in the early stages of rehabilitative programs or those who have no access to assistance. The project objective is to develop a client data tracking system that will be used to prove the economic and social value of long-term stroke rehabilitation. The hypothesis to be tested is that stroke victims who use the Stroke Recovery Center are less of a financial burden on the health and social service budgets than those who do not access Stroke Recovery Center services. The Stroke Recovery Center, as the best practice model for continuing care for stroke survivors, requires eligibility for predictable and sustainable funding from government, private insurance, and/or medical group providers to be replicated in other locations.

Research Design and Parameters

We have collected and tabulated data from 95 clients who, as of February 1, 2008, were Stroke Recovery Center users, having been there 3+ months and attended at least 3 times per month or more. In year 2, we collected data on 119 clients that met the ongoing criteria and were able to compare their data to each other as in the first study as well as to the data collected in year 1.

The initial baseline data was analyzed using the criteria of length of attendance (LOS) at the Stroke Recovery Center. Looking at the year 2 data, we found that the length of attendance remained a median of 2 years with the heaviest concentration continuing to be in the 2- and 3-year time frame consistent with the year 1 data.

Having two years of data, we were able to track the dropout rate and analyze the characteristics of those who do not continue and reasons for noncompliance with the program along with the utilization criteria we determined in the year 1 study.

With the median LOS at 2 years, data points were again compared to determine if there were differences in the early users as compared to those who have been at the center for 2+ years. With that data in hand, analysis went deeper to look at the changes from year 1 as well.

Results

The data findings were addressed and compared to data from year 1 in the following categories:

Client dropout in year 2. This category was identified as clients who had attended at least 3 months in 2008 but had dropped out by December of 2008. There was a 17% dropout as a percentage of the whole; however, of that number, 61% were from death and/or deteriorating health issues that no longer allowed the client to participate. The other reasons reported were dissatisfaction, transportation, and graduation reasons.

Age and sex of clients. The average age of clients attending grew older slightly over 3 years. The median age is 72, up two years from year 1. The largest increase is in the group of clients who have attended over 2 years with an average of 73.6 years and a median of 75 years. The age range in the year 2 study group was from 25 years of age to 92 years of age, which helps to explain the differential. The client base continues to reflect national norms with men growing from 53% of the total to 62% of the total after the 2-year average.

Prescription drug usage. The average number of drugs taken by the client population grew by 1 and 0.8 respectively per day to 5.5 in the group participating under 2 years and 5.3 in the group participating over 2 years. Median drug usage was 5 for each group. While this is a positive move in those attending longer, correlation appears to follow comorbidities and age as opposed to time spent. However, the positive move toward less drug usage will continue to be followed to determine if the drug education along with the general well-being of the client base may have influence as they stay longer in the programs.

Ambulation. While the year 1 data indicated a difference in ambulation and ambulation aids, showing a movement from walkers to canes among those who spend a longer time at the center than from those that are in the first 2 years, year 2 data is less clear. The decline in walker use may be shifted to cane, but also there is a significant increase in wheelchair usage, suggesting that more clients may be requiring greater assistance as time goes on. However, the year 2 data also suggests that more clients are being moved to ambulation assistance. This may be related to the increased age of the group reported and/or more clinical analysis of client need related to the results of the first-year study. It is less conclusive that length of time at the center is a major influence on ambulation.

Orthotics. Orthotics usage is showing a stronger decline than in the year 1 data indicated. Of those in their first year at the center, 51% are using orthotics. By the time they have spent 2 years at the center, 29.2% are using orthotics. The biggest drop occurs after the first year at the center.

Transportation. The reliance on families and caregivers for transportation to the center increased in the year 2 data to 67.6% and declining to 41.2% after the clients have been at the center for 2 years. The change to using the bus for transportation grows from 5.9% to 29.4%. However, of great interest is the percentage of clients who take the bus after the first year—24.4%. This number is higher than was shown in our first study. Of the dropouts who cited transportation as an issue, 3 of 5 were dependent upon families.

Emergency room visits. Over year 2, there is further reduction in the ER visits by the clients who have been at the center for more than two years. Overall, 25% of the client population visited the ER in 2008. Of those who have been at the center more than 2 years, only 12.2% visited the ER while 35% of the clients who have been at the center less than two years visited the ER. These results exceed the prior results and offer an even greater savings to the health-care system as a whole.

Falls. There has been an overall reduction in the percentage of the population who suffer falls to 20.4% as opposed to 30% in year 1 of the study. As clients are at the center 2+ years, that percentage is reduced to 18.4%. There is a drop after the 2+ year mark while the difference between year 1 and year 2 at the center is negligible.

Conclusions

There are positive changes in the direction and velocity of outcomes that are noted in the data from year 2. The major variable that has changed is the study itself and its reported results that may be causing a Hawthorne effect both on the part of the client themselves who know the utilization points that are being reported upon and the staff therapists who have read the results and want to improve upon what was reported in year 1. The move to riding the bus showing such an increase would fall into this category, as would ER visits, falls, and use of orthotics. That said, the results of the program become even more important in demonstrating cost savings for the health-care system as a whole and supporting even more strongly the introduction of this program to stroke survivors and their families throughout the country.

ORGANIZATIONAL HEALTH INITIATIVE PROJECT

Introduction

The Organizational Health Initiative Project (OHIP) is now in its second year of data gathering and analysis. The OHIP methodology is to gather data regarding outcomes of treatment for chronic stroke suffers from the existing patient base and compare such data to stroke victims who are in the early stages of rehabilitative programs or those who have not access to assistance. The project objective is to develop a client data tracking system that will be used to prove the economic and social value of long-term stroke rehabilitation. The hypothesis to be tested is that stroke victims who use the Stroke Recovery Center are less of a financial burden on the health and social service budgets than those who do not access Stroke Recovery Center services. Stroke Recovery Center, as the best practice model for continuing care for stroke survivors, requires eligibility for predictable and sustainable funding from government, private insurance, and/or medical group providers to be replicated in other locations.

RESEARCH DESIGN AND PARAMETERS

Design

We have collected and tabulated data from 95 clients who, as of February 1, 2008, were Stroke Recovery Center users, having been there 3+ months and attended at least 3 times per month or more. In year 2, we collected data on 119 clients that met the ongoing criteria and were able to compare their data to each other as in the first study as well as to the data collected in year 1.

The initial baseline data was analyzed using the criteria of length of attendance (LOS) at the Stroke Recovery Center. Looking at the year 2 data, we found that the length of attendance remained a median of 2 years with the heaviest concentration continuing to be in the 2- and 3-year time frame consistent with the year 1 data.

Having two years of data, we were able to track the dropout rate and analyze the characteristics of those who do not continue and reasons for noncompliance with the program along with the utilization criteria we determined in the year 1 study.

With the median LOS at 2 years, data points were again compared to determine if there were differences in the early users as compared to those who have been at the center for 2+ years. With that data in hand, analysis went deeper to look at the changes from year 1 as well.

Parameters

The baseline data is analyzed using the criteria of length of attendance (LOS) to the center to keep the results and outcomes consistent for analysis. This parameter was chosen to determine if clients show improvement over time spent at the center and partaking in the programs. To support this as the supporting factor to recovery, the data was also analyzed and adjusted for age variations, comorbidities, type of stroke, and length of time since the last stroke. The year 2 data was also rigorously examined to ensure that the results were consistent.

The 119 clients in the year 2 group have an average (mean) length of attendance at the center of 2.6 years with a median of 2 years. The spread continues to be great, so the use of the median has greater validity. The median is the middle of the data set and has an equal number of data points above and below the median value. Therefore, going forward with our analysis as we did with the year 1 data, we will use the median number of 2 years attendance and compare the greater than (>) 2 year attendees to the less than (<) 2 year attendees. We did, however, add to some of the outcomes that we measured a further analysis looking at the first year compared to the 1+ years.

Further, we had the ability to look at the dropout clients and analyze that cohort and its effect both on the data and on the treatment modalities. The dropout percentage was 17% (26 clients) of the total for 2008. Of that, 26% (7 clients) died and 34% (9 clients) were unable to attend because of deteriorating health. Of that group, 50% were in their first year at the center. Two out of three dissatisfied clients were also in their first year while the third is a client who has been coming to the center off and on for 20 years, having had a stroke as a young woman and never recovering her ability to talk. Our two graduates, no longer in need of services, were here 5 years and less than 1 year; however, the latter was a TBI as opposed to a stroke survivor. Those identifying transportation as an issue (5 clients) varied in attendance from 11 years to -1 years.

We looked at the following data based on the client's length of attendance to compare it to the prior year's results:

- Age and sex
- Transportation
- Comorbidities and drug usage
- Ambulation
- Orthotic usage
- ER visits
- Number of falls

RESULTS

Age and Sex of Clients

The average age of clients attending in year 1 was 68 years of age with a median of 70 years of age. Year 2 showed an increase in the average and the median ages, 71.2 and 72 respectively. However, the age range in the second year expanded to 25 to 92. We had two clients in their nineties join us in 2008, and that does skew the data upward. The single client in his twenties was a TBI as opposed to a stroke.

The year 1 group that had attended less than 2 years had a mean age of 67 with the median 68 years of age. The year 2 data aged this group to 69.3 average and 71 median with a standard deviation of 12.2. This reflects the very elderly clients who joined us along with the very young. In the first year, the group that had attended longer than 2 years was older with an average (mean) age of 70.6 years of age and a median age of 71 years. In year 2 data, the average grew to 73.6 and the median to 75. The standard deviation was 10.9, still reflecting a wide range of ages. Results do not correlate to age differentials, suggesting that improvements that are made are not age dependent.

Ages of the dropout group do not correlate with the reported issue. Deaths range from 47 as the youngest to 88 as the eldest, an average of 70.6 and a median of 73 with a standard deviation of 12.6. Those in declining health were older with an average of 72.2, median of 74, and a standard deviation of 11.1, ranging from 53 to 87. The graduates, those expressing that they no longer needed the services of the center, were 42 and 25, well below the average and median ages.

The gender of the client base that stays at the center over 2 years is higher than the national norms with regard to the percentage of females treated. In the first two years, the percentage is closer to the national norm of 43% of strokes each year.

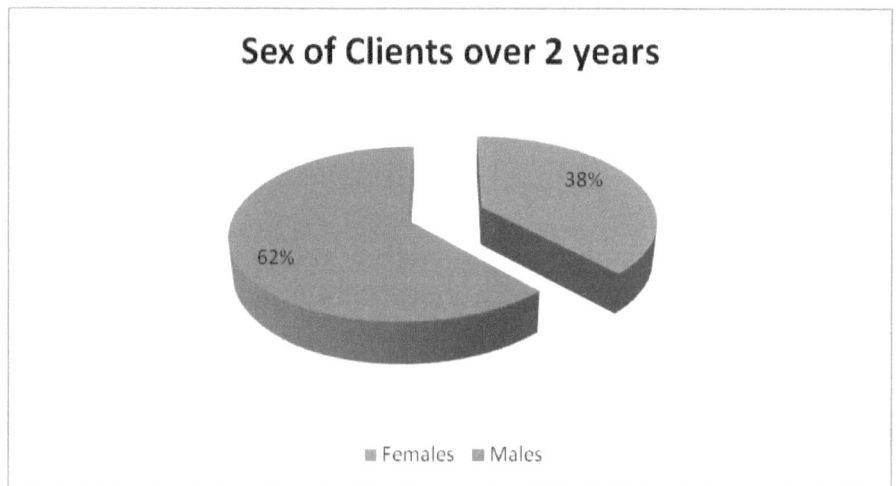

Among the clients who have attended less than 2 years in year 1, the numbers were almost equal: 49% women and 51% men. In year 2 data, there were fewer females (47%) and more males (53%), which is slightly ahead of the national norms. For those who have been here longer than 2 years, the percentage changed in the first year to 35% women and 65% men, while in year 2 of the study there were 38% females and 62% males.

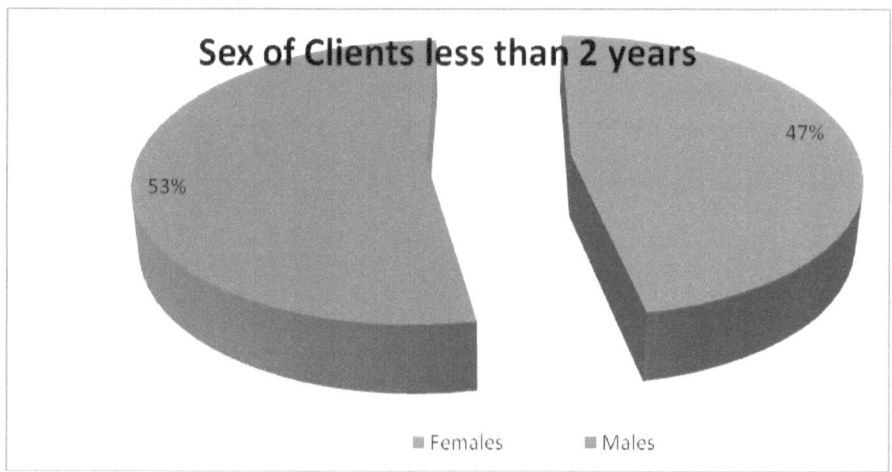

Females account for 61% of the deaths from stroke each year. In the dropout group, deaths were 4 females and 3 males. Of interest is the fact that the 3 males who died did so in their first year at the center while the females who died had been at the center over 2+ years. Those in declining health were 4 females and 5 males. Males and females were evenly distributed in the dissatisfied and transportation group; however, both our graduates were male.

Prescription Drug Usage

The average (mean) number of drugs taken by the client population in the year 1 study was 4.5 per day with a median of 5 and standard deviation of 3 that indicated a number of significant outliers that are attributable to comorbidities. In the second year, the average increased to 5.5 in those with less than two years at the center and 2.3 for those who have been at the center longer. The median numbers are both 5, which is the same as it was in year 1 of the study. With the range being high, the initial presumption that the number of drugs and usage appears to be more highly related to the comorbidities than to the years spent at the center. The consistency of the data supports this contention.

Transportation

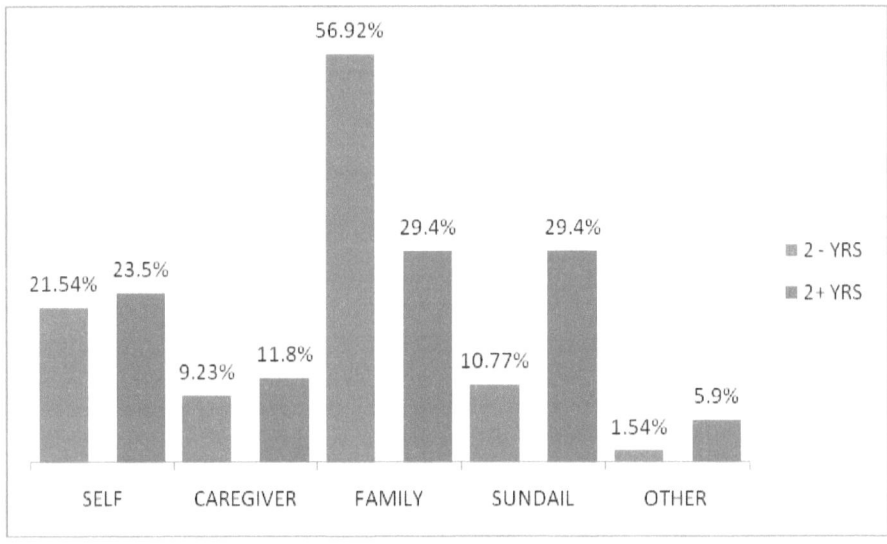

As was true with the year 1 data, the shift to public and/or commercial forms of transportation away from reliance on the family is noticeable after the clients have been at the center for 2+ years. In the early years, 65.1% of clients rely on their families or caregivers for transportation needs while that percentage shrinks to 41.2% after year 2. Those taking public transportation grows from 12.3% to 36.3%. The constancy of caregiver transport is probably due to the need for assistance both for transportation and for participation at the center.

Among the five clients that cited transportation as a reason for discontinuing their therapy, three were dependent upon their families while the other two used commercial methods. The data in this area is inconclusive.

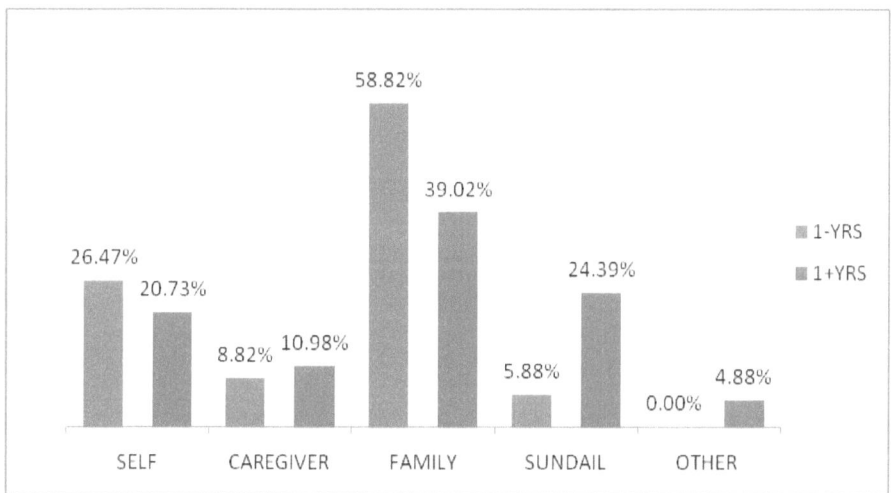

Of interest in analysis of the data is the shift that occurs after the first year of attendance. This may be one of the areas that we are seeing some of the Hawthorne effect. The results of the first study may be incentivizing both the staff therapists and the clients to work harder and to show results more quickly since the shift to commercial transportation is so dramatic even after one year in reducing the reliance on families and increasing independence.

Ambulation

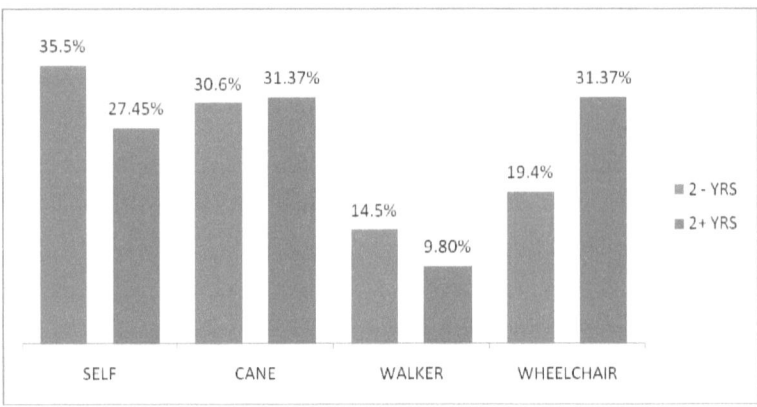

While the year 1 data indicated a difference in ambulation and ambulation aids, showing a movement from walkers to canes among those who spend a longer time at the center than from those that are in the first 2 years, year 2 data is less clear. The decline in walker use may be shifting to cane but also may be shifting to wheelchairs as there is a significant increase in wheelchair usage, suggesting that more clients may be requiring greater assistance as time goes on. The year 2 data suggests that, overall, more clients are being moved to ambulation assistance than was the case in the first year of the study. Looking at the movement that is occurring after the first year of attendance, the data suggests that therapists are moving clients to more ambulation assistance at an early stage in their program. This may be related to the increased age of the group reported and/or more clinical analysis of client need related to the results of the first-year study. It is less conclusive that the length of time at the center is a major influence on ambulation assistance.

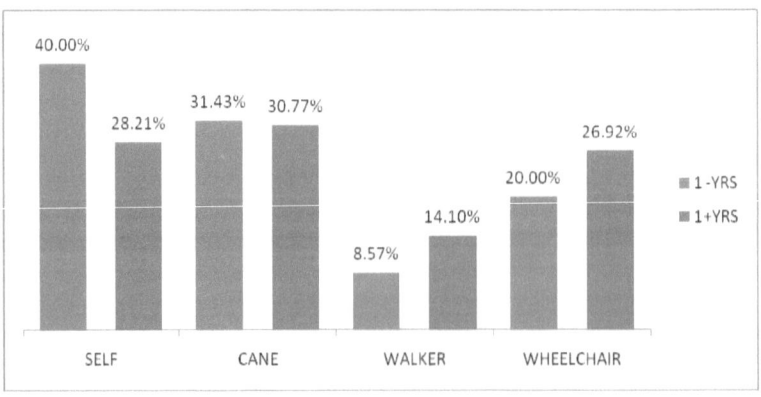

Orthotics

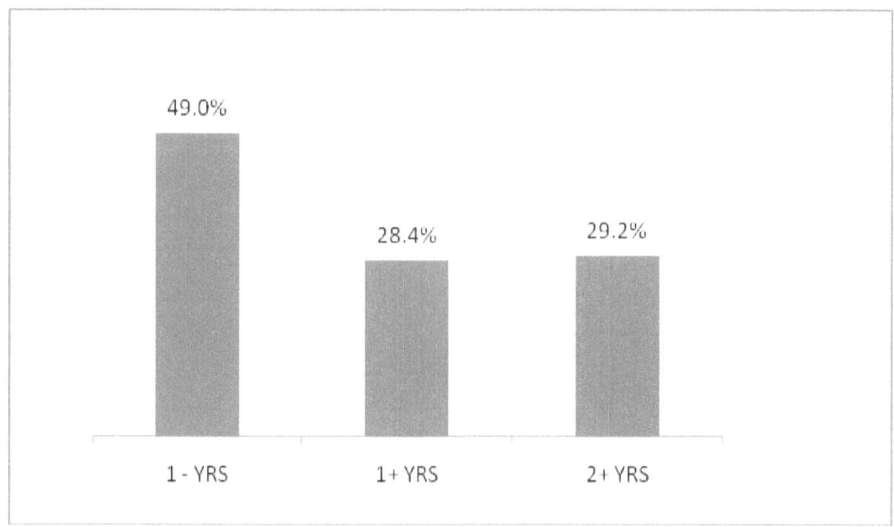

Use of orthotics for ambulation assistance by clients increased from the data from year 1 of the study in those who have attended the center for more than two years to 29.2% from 21%. Additionally, the number of clients who initially used orthotic support increased to 49% from 32%. The presentation of clients who are using orthotics may be attributed in part to the increase in age; however, a significant drop in usage occurs after the first year of attendance and is stable thereafter. These results may be in part attributed to the Hawthorne effect on both the staff therapists as well as the clients themselves. Attention of appropriate supports in conjunction with the changed results in ambulation assistance seem to support that attention is being given at an earlier stage of recovery. The supposition is more credible than an improvement of overall recovery results because of the factor of advanced age that would tend to move the data to a longer recovery. The follow-up years will prove to be interesting in indicating which supposition is correct.

Emergency Room Visits

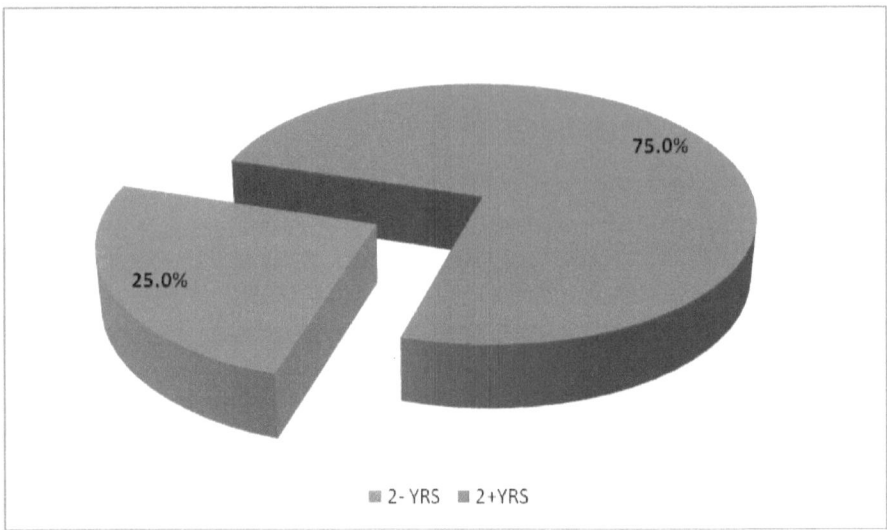

In 2008, 25% of the client population made at least one visit to an ER, which was less than the 32% of clients from the year prior. Use of the ER declined from 35% among those who were in the first two years of attendance to 25% among those who have attended more than two years. The first year of the study showed 13% of clients who have been at the center more than 2 years used the ER while the year 2 data showed 12.2% of clients had a visit to the ER. These results are consistent from year to year and support continued recovery of health and well-being with attendance at the center.

Cost for ER visits continues to be a major drain on the health-care system as a whole. The ability to successfully have an influence on reducing this cost supports the inclusion of the therapies designed and provided at the Stroke Recovery Center to long-term care programs for stroke survivors throughout the country.

Falls

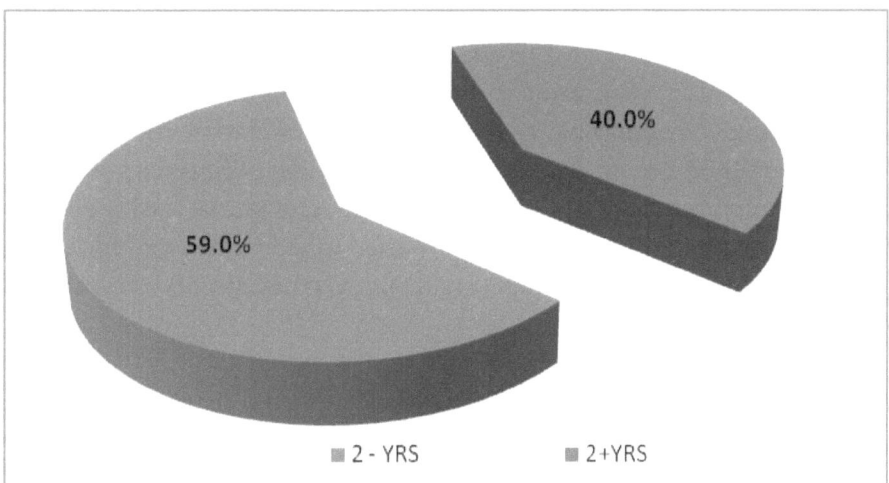

There was an overall reduction in the number of clients who suffered falls in 2008 with 20.4% of the client base reporting falls as opposed to 30% the year prior. This current number is well below the national norm for seniors. Considering the client base is elderly and handicapped, the numbers show significant progress in treatment. This is a statistic that may be influenced by the Hawthorne affect along with the ambulation and orthotics. Looking at data of clients who have attended more than 2 years, falls are reduced by 19% over the clients who are in their first 2 years of attendance. The clients that have been with the center less than 2 years suffered falls at nearly double the rate of those who have been at the center longer. Data that compares clients in their first year of attendance show 54% of falls occur in that first year as compared to 45% in the years afterward. This supports the contention that the staff therapists are having a greater influence on the physical recovery of clients, particularly when the advanced age of the client base is factored in.

The cost reductions to the health-care system as a whole from reduction of falls in the frail and elderly is significant not only in the medical cost, the hospital cost, and the medication cost but also in elements like first-responder cost and lost productivity of caregivers needed for recovery. This statistic by itself supports the inclusion of the therapies of the center in a long-term care plan for stroke survivors throughout the country.

CONCLUSIONS

There are some positive changes in the outcomes that are noted from the data in year 2. The major variable that has changed is the study itself and its reported results that may be causing something of a Hawthorne effect both on the part of the client themselves who know the utilization points that are being reported upon and the staff therapists who have read the results and want to improve upon what was reported in year 1. The move to riding the bus showing such an increase would fall into this category, as would ER visits, falls, and use of orthotics.

The value of the center as a functional intervention in the continuum of care for stroke survivors continues to be supported by the data for transportation usage, orthotics, emergency room visits, and falls. Reduction of incidents along with ambulation supports and moving to independent use of transportation all translate to dollar savings for the health-care system as well as reducing cost to the economy as a whole by reducing productivity loss from those family members who provide care for long-term stroke survivors.

On the other hand, it continues to be important to note that a correlation between the amount of time spent at the Stroke Recovery Center and improvement in the numbers is not statistically significant. In other words, we are unable to say neither that the longer one stays with the program, the better he/she will be, nor are we able to say that the program causes less falls, lowers emergency room usage, etc. Further, we are also unable to correlate these improvements to age, type of stroke, passage of time since the stroke, or comorbidities. By eliminating linear regression of the possible causative elements, we are left with the common factor variation that is most significant being the time spent in the program with one's peer group as having the greatest influence on recovery as measured by these parameters. Taking the advancing age of the individual as he/she continues to attend the center, the results we have posted become even more significant. It is possible to posit that, while unable to support a linear relationship, we are able to demonstrate recovery and maintenance of improvement as the client continues to age. This outcome is of high value to the elderly population.

Year 2 data continues to support our position and our credibility as the best practice for long-term rehabilitation for stroke survivors.

STROKE RECOVERY CENTER

Update to

Organizational Health Initiative Project

December 2009

Prepared August 2010

Funding provided by the Desert Healthcare District

CONTENTS

1. Executive Summary 149

2. Organizational Health Initiative Project 153

3. Research Design and Parameters 154

4. Results 157
   a. Age and Sex of Clients 157
   b. Prescription Drug Usage 159
   c. Transportation 160
   d. Ambulation 161
   e. Orthotics 162
   f. Emergency Room Visits 163
   g. Falls 164

5. Conclusions 165

EXECUTIVE SUMMARY

Organizational Health Initiative Project

The Organizational Health Initiative Project (OHIP) is now in its third year of data gathering and analysis. The OHIP methodology is to gather data regarding outcomes of treatment for chronic stroke and TBI sufferers from the existing patient base and compare such data to stroke and TBI victims and survivors along with national data regarding seniors and disabled populations. The project objective has been to develop a client data tracking system that will be used to prove the economic and social value of long-term stroke rehabilitation. The hypothesis tested is that stroke and TBI victims who use the Stroke Recovery Center are less of a financial burden on the health and social service budgets than those who do not have access to Stroke Recovery Center services. The Stroke Recovery Center, as the best practice model for continuing care for stroke survivors, requires eligibility for predictable and sustainable funding from government, private insurance, and/or medical group providers to become sustainable, to develop more comprehensive programming, and to be replicated in other locations. The project is designed to provide the value proposition to potential funders within the health-care system and position the center as a value-added partner in care.

Research Design and Parameters

We have collected and tabulated data from 89 clients who, as of January 1, 2009, were Stroke Recovery Center users, having been there 3+ months and attended at least 3 times per month or more. We were able to compare the data points with the cohorts we collected in years 1 and 2.

The initial baseline data was analyzed using the criteria of length of attendance (LOS) at the Stroke Recovery Center. Looking at the year 3 data, we found that the length of attendance remained a median of 2 years with the heaviest concentration continuing to be in the 2- and 3-year time frame consistent with the year 1 and 2 data.

Having three years of data, we were able to track the dropout rate and analyze the characteristics of those who do not continue and reasons for noncompliance with the program along with the utilization criteria we determined in the year 1 and 2 study.

With the median LOS at 2 years, data points were again compared to determine if there were differences in the early users as compared to those who have been at the center for 2+ years. With that data in hand, analysis went deeper to look at the changes from year 1 and 2 as well.

Results

The data findings were addressed and compared to data from year 1 and 2 in the following categories:

Client dropout in year 2. This category was identified as clients who had attended at least 3 months in 2009 but had dropped out by December of 2009. There was an 11.2% dropout as a percentage of the whole; however, of that number, 44.6% were from death and/or deteriorating health issues that no longer allowed the client to participate. The other reasons reported were moving out of the area, return to work, and no reason.

Age and sex of clients. The average age of clients was 68.8, similar to the first year of the study. The median age is 69, slightly lower than year 2. As expected, the group that has a longer LOS has a slightly higher average age of 71.8. The client base continues to reflect national norms with the highest propensity for stoke being in the 60–79 age group and men and women being at equal risk. As the group ages, men become higher risk, but prior to 60 years of age, women have almost 2 times the risk over men. This is supported by our sex differentials—a higher propensity of women in the first 2 years, but the men catching up as the LOS extends.

Prescription drug usage. Prescription drug usage per patient increased in year 3 to 7 per patient. This is in line with the Kaiser study of seniors that identifies 7 as the norm. Examining the drugs indicate a wide variety of drugs used, including dietary supplements and vitamin usage. Comorbidities appear to be the major determining factor and suggest that drug usage needs to be examined on a case-by-case basis.

Transportation. The shift to public and/or commercial forms of transportation and a return to self-transportation continue to support the rehabilitation efforts to increase confidence and independence and decrease reliance on family. Professional caregivers as transporters remain constant. Bus usage moved from 5.3% in the first 2 years to 20% in the over-2-years group.

Ambulation. Year 3 data indicates that there is a continued aggressive move to utilize mobility aids among the patients. Initial data seemed to indicate that there would be less use of support aids as the years went on; however, the data suggests the opposite is true. Stability and balance are critical to successful mobility, and independence and the use of aids does aid that process.

Orthotics. Initially, it was contended that orthotic use would decline as the years progress, but as with ambulation aid, the use of orthotics has increased as the years progress. This suggests that orthotics use is being prescribed to increase balance and mobility in an aggressive manner and should be correlated to reduction in falls.

Emergency room visits. In 2009, 17.3% of the patients made at least one visit to an emergency room (ER), even less than the prior years. All these visits came from the group who has been at the center less than 2 years. As the patients remain at the center, the propensity to use the ER declines, which offers significant savings to the health-care system.

Falls. The percentage of patients who fall has declined each year of the study to 13.5% in year 3. This number is well below the national average for seniors of 30%. The increased use of ambulation aids and orthotics can be correlated to this as the concentration on balance and strengthening used individually in the exercise-therapy program can be cited as supporting these numbers.

Conclusions

The data has strongly supported the efforts of the Stroke Recovery Center but suggests that the center is only taking the first steps to assist their patients on their recovery. The data supports the creation of an environment in which healing can take place and where patients can gain some control over their lives, regaining some of the skills and independence they enjoyed prior to the stroke or TBI. The data further supports the value of exercise in increasing secure mobility that in turn adds to confidence and independence. However, on the other hand, the data also suggests that patient-focused care should be instituted to maximize value for each individual patient. Cost savings to the system should be allocated to support this case management and program development and need to be garnered from the sources that benefit. There are clear and undeniable data to support this notion, and it is the clear direction that the studies have revealed.

ORGANIZATIONAL HEALTH INITIATIVE PROJECT

Introduction

The Organizational Health Initiative Project (OHIP) is now in its third year of data gathering and analysis. The OHIP methodology is to gather data regarding outcomes of treatment for chronic stroke sufferers from the existing patient base and compare such data to stroke victims who may or may not have access to assistance and to norms provided for other chronic disease sufferers, elderly, and frail populations. The project has developed a client data tracking system that is being used to prove the economic and social value of long-term stroke rehabilitation. The hypothesis to be tested is that stroke victims who use the Stroke Recovery Center are less of a financial burden on the health and social service budgets than those who do not access Stroke Recovery Center services. Quantification of the cost/benefit lends precision to the reasoning for long-term rehabilitation to be a functional part of the continuum of care. The Stroke Recovery Center, as the best practice model for continuing care for stroke survivors, is currently ineligible for sustainable funding and, as such, is at high risk for failure. Cost-benefit analysis is being used to present the case for eligibility for predictable and sustainable funding from government, private insurance, and/or medical group providers to be replicated in other locations.

RESEARCH DESIGN AND PARAMETERS

Design

We have collected and tabulated data from 89 clients who, as of January 1, 2009, were Stroke Recovery Center users, having been there 3+ months and attended at least 3 times per month or more and participated in at least two of the rehabilitation modalities offered at the center. Those who just participate in speech therapy or just in exercise therapy are not included in this comprehensive study. In year 3, we collected data on 89 clients that met this ongoing criteria and were able to compare their data to each other as in the first study as well as to the data collected in years 1 and 2.

The initial baseline data was analyzed using the criteria of length of attendance (LOS) at the Stroke Recovery Center. Looking at the year 3 data, we found that the length of attendance remained a median of 2 years with the heaviest concentration continuing to be in the 2- and 3-year time frame consistent with the year 1 and 2 data. The average LOS was 3.4 years, but the spread was from 15 years to the minimum of 3 months required for inclusion in the study.

Having three years of data, we were able to track the dropout rate and analyze the characteristics of those who do not continue and reasons for noncompliance with the program along with the utilization criteria we determined in the year 1 and 2 study.

With the median LOS at 2 years, data points were again compared to determine if there were differences in the early users as compared to those who have been at the center for 2+ years. With that data in hand, analysis went deeper to look at the changes from year 1 and 2 as well.

Parameters

The baseline data is analyzed using the criteria of length of attendance (LOS) to the center to keep the results and outcomes consistent for analysis. This parameter was chosen to determine if clients show improvement over time spent at the center and partaking in the programs. To support this as the major contributing factor to recovery, the data was also analyzed and adjusted for age variations, comorbidities, type of stroke, and length of time since the last stroke. The year 3 data was also rigorously examined to ensure that the results were consistent.

The 89 clients in the year 3 group have an average (mean) length of attendance at the center of 3.4 years with a median of 2 years. This is a significantly higher average than last year primarily due to the longevity of a number of our patients who have over 10 years attendance. The spread is between 15 years and 3 months, so the use of the median has greater validity. The median is the middle of the data set and has an equal number of data points above and below the median value. Therefore, going forward with our analysis as we did with the year 1 and 2 data, we will use the median number of 2 years attendance and compare the greater than (>) 2 year attendees to the less than (<) 2 year attendees. In our second year, we added to some of the outcomes that we measured a further analysis, looking at the first year compared to the 1+ years. As appropriate, we did the same in year 3.

Further, we had the ability to look at the dropout clients and analyze that cohort and its effect both on the data and on the treatment modalities. The dropout percentage was 11.2% for year 3, a total of 10 patients. This is compared to 17% (26 patients) of the total for 2008. Of that 11.2%, 30% (3 patients) died compared to 26% (7 patients) the year prior. Patients that were transferred to other facility's care or were unable to attend due to deteriorating health totaled 40% in year 3, a bit higher than the 34% (9 patients) from the year prior. We also had one patient who moved out of the area, one client who was able to go back to his volunteer job, and one patient who left but has a history of taking a few years off and then returning. In terms of trends, we are seeing a core group of survivors who take part in all the services but extensive growth in specialty services of speech and exercise.

We looked at the following data based on the client's length of attendance to compare it to the prior year's results:

- Age and sex
- Transportation

- Comorbidities and drug usage
- Ambulation
- Orthotic usage
- ER visits
- Number of falls

RESULTS

Age and Sex of Clients

The average age of clients attending in year 1 was 68 years of age with a median of 70 years of age. Year 2 showed an increase in the average and the median ages, 71.2 and 72 respectively. However, the age range in the second year expanded to 25 to 92. In year 3, the average age was 68.8 years of age with a median age of 69 with only one client in her nineties remaining with us.

The year 1 group that had attended less than 2 years had a mean age of 67 with the median 68 years of age. The year 2 data aged this group to 69.3 average and 71 median with a standard deviation of 12.2. Year 3 has an average of 65.3 years of age but with a standard deviation of 16.2, indicating the wide spread of ages. In the first year, the group that had attended longer than 2 years was older with an average (mean) age of 70.6 years of age and a median age of 71 years. In year 2 data, the average grew to 73.6 and the median to 75. The standard deviation was 10.9. In year 3, the average was 71.8 with a standard deviation of 10.9.

The consistency to the ages of the groups, even with the high level of age deviation resulting from the few TBI patients who tend to be under 40 years of age, suggests that tolerance for rehabilitation is highest among the 60–79 years of age cohort. This group has a prevalence of stroke of 7.4 to 7.5% of the population, much less than the 80+ group.

Deaths range from 47 as the youngest to 88 as the eldest in our year 2 results, while in year 3, we had one death at 89 years of age with the other two in their early seventies. There was little in age correlation to suggest age-related comorbidity problems or moving away from the center.

The gender of the client base that stays at the center over 2 years in year 3 lowered from a high level of 62% males to 54.2% males. Incidence of stroke in males prior to age 60 is higher than for females, but tends to even out in the 60–69 age group and increases again in the 80+ group. Since the group that stays with us tends to be older, the trends all follow the national norms.

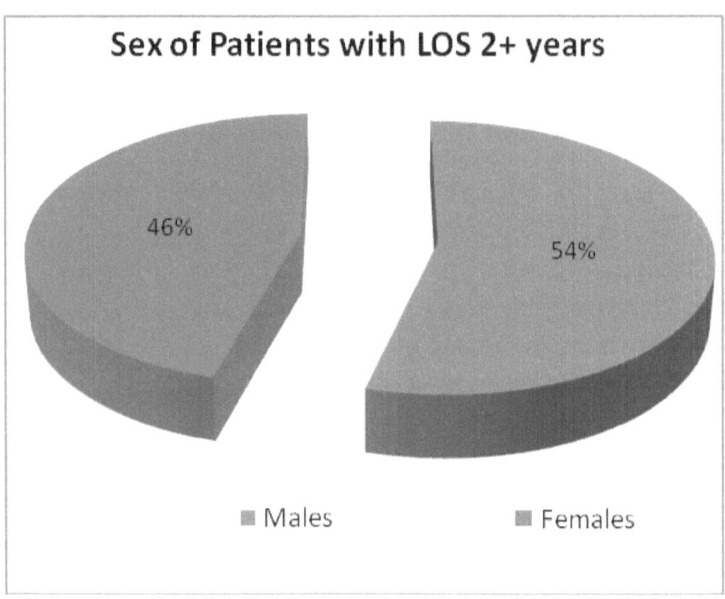

Among the clients who have attended less than 2 years in year 1, the numbers were almost equal: 49% women and 51% men. In year 2 data, there were fewer females (47%) and more males (53%), which is slightly ahead of the national norms. For those who have been here longer than 2 years, the percentage changed in the first year to 35% women and 65% men. While in year 2 of the study, there were 38% females and 62% males. Year 3 shows a reverse with only 46.3% being males and 53.7% being females. Women in the 40–59 years of age group tend to have strokes at a much higher percentage of the population than do men—2.7% compared to 1.0% for men.

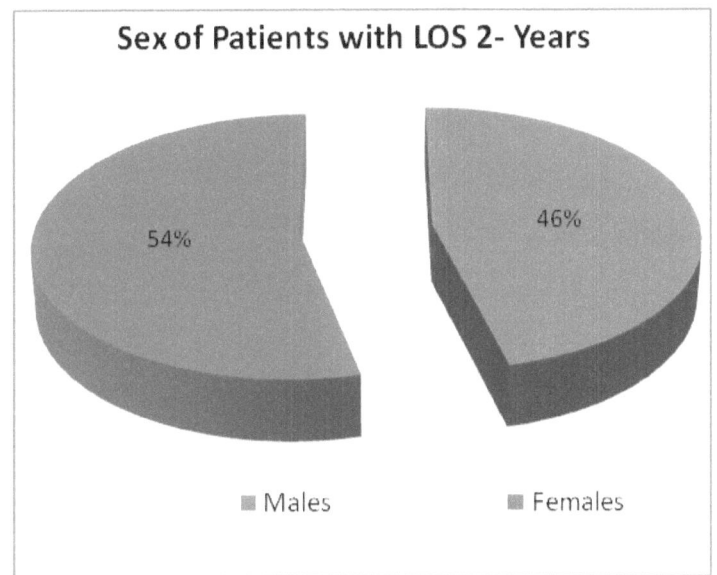

Females account for 61% of the deaths from stroke each year. In the dropout group, deaths were all females, one of who had just started with us but was 89 years of age. There is no correlation to age with those who suffer comorbidities or moved to other areas.

Prescription Drug Usage

The average (mean) number of drugs taken by the client population in the year 1 study was 4.5 per day with a median of 5 and standard deviation of 3, which indicated a number of significant outliers that are attributable to comorbidities. In the second year, the average increased to 5.5 in those with less than two years at the center and 2.3 for those who have been at the center longer. The median numbers are both 5, which is the same as it was in year 1 of the study. With the range being high, the initial presumption that the number of drugs and usage appears to be more highly related to the comorbidities than to the years spent at the center. The consistency of the data supports this contention.

Year 3 data confirms earlier data. The average number of drugs taken is 7.1, consistent with the Kaiser study of senior drug usage. Drug usage does not vary with the time spent at the center but does vary significantly with comorbidities.

Transportation

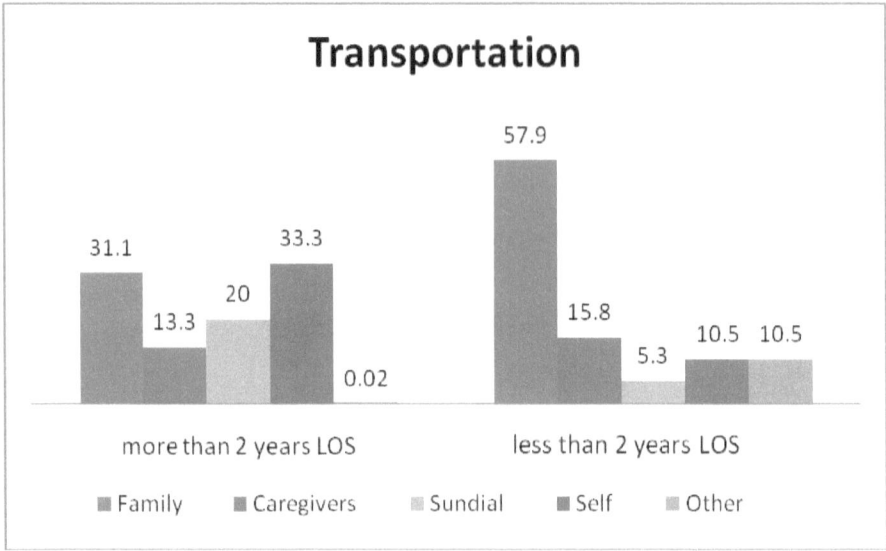

As was true with the year 1 and year 2 data, the shift to public and/or commercial forms of transportation away from reliance on the family is noticeable after the clients have been at the center for 2+ years. In the early years, 73.7% of patients rely on their families or caregivers for transportation needs while that percentage shrinks to 44.4% after being with us for 2+ years. Those taking public transportation grows from 5.3% to 20.0%. The constancy of caregivers decreases very little over time, probably due to the need for assistance both for transportation and for participation at the center.

Clients able to bring themselves to the center increases after the first 2 years of attendance from 10.5% to 33.5%.

We did not see the significant increase we saw in year 2 after the first year, suggesting that the first year's results are more replicable over the long-term and, therefore, have a higher degree of validity.

Ambulation

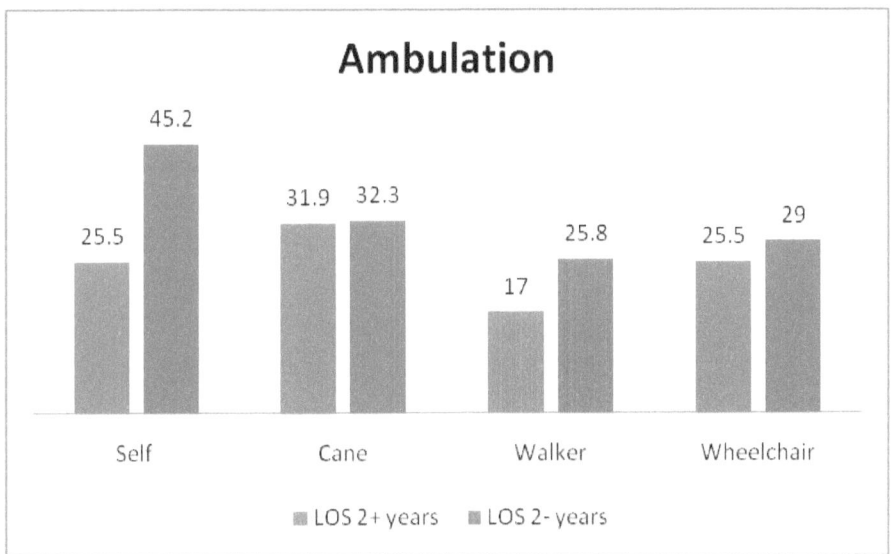

While the year 1 data indicated a difference in ambulation and ambulation aids, showing a movement from walkers to canes among those who spend a longer time at the center than from those that are in the first 2 years, year 2 data is less clear. The decline in walker use may be shifting to cane but also may be shifting to wheelchairs as there is a significant increase in wheelchair usage, suggesting that more clients may be requiring greater assistance as time goes on. The year 2 data suggests that, overall, more clients are being moved to ambulation assistance than was the case in the first year of the study. Looking at the movement that is occurring after the first year of attendance, the data suggests that therapists are moving clients to more ambulation assistance at an early stage in their program. This may be related to the increased age of the group reported and/or more clinical analysis of client need related to the results of the first-year study.

The results from year 2 are upheld as we move into year 3. We see a big move from self-ambulation in uses of canes and walkers. Wheelchair usage remains somewhat constant. This suggests the correlation is to the age and comorbidities of the population along with therapists moving patients to assisted mobility to support balance and stability in their homes and in the center.

Orthotics

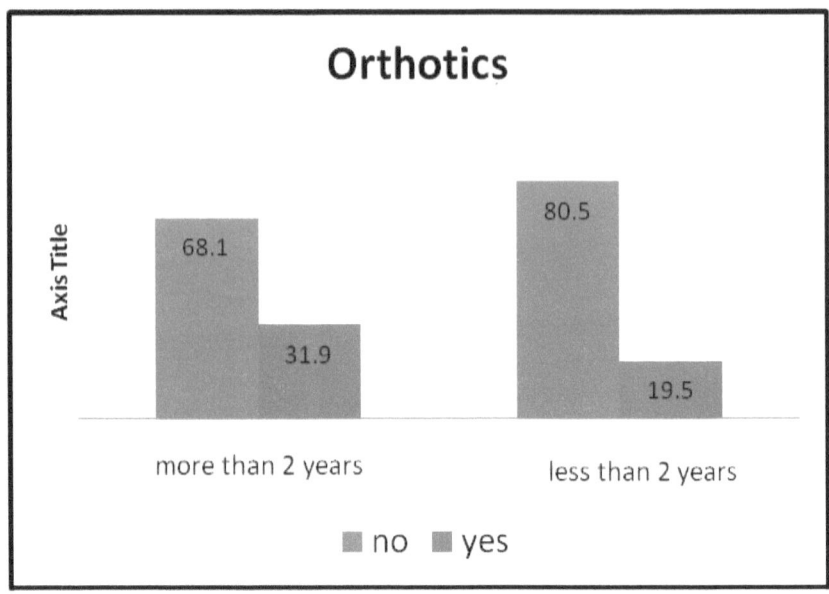

Use of orthotics for ambulation assistance by clients increased from the data from year 1 of the study in those who have attended the center for more than two years to 29.2% from 21%. Additionally, the number of clients who initially used orthotic support increased to 49% from 32%. Last year, the data indicated that patients' increased use of orthotics may be attributed in part to the increase in age; however, attention to appropriate supports in conjunction with the changed results in ambulation assistance seem to support that more attention is being given to the benefits of extra support. All 80.5% of new patients are not using orthotic support when they start with the center. By year 2+, 68.1% of patients are not using support while 31.9% of patients are using orthotics for support and help in ambulation, suggesting that more patients are being assisted by orthotic supports as they are given more rehabilitation.

Emergency Room Visits

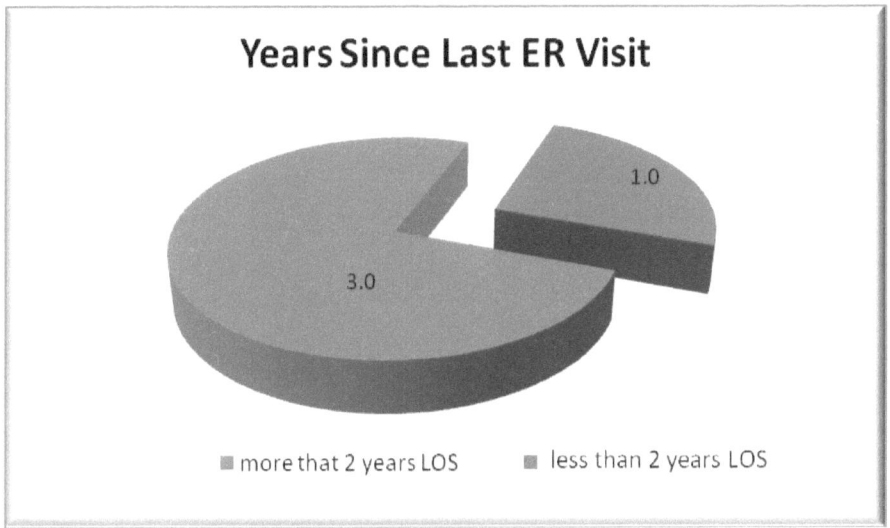

In 2009, 17.3% of the patients made at least one visit to an emergency room, down from 25% and 32% of the patient populations in the years prior. All the visits in 2009 were recorded by the group who had been at the center in their first 2 years. This being the case, looking at the years since the last visit to the ER by the different cohorts gives us a better picture of predictive behavior correlated to the time spent at the center. Patients that have more than 2 years LOS have not visited an ER for 3 years (median) while those with less than 2 years LOS have only 1 year since their last visit to the ER. While the early joining group comes to the center an average of 2.1 years after their stroke and, therefore, possibly would have a more current ER experience, as they remain at the center, they are less likely to seek emergency care.

Cost for ER visits continues to be a major drain on the health-care system as a whole. The ability to successfully have an influence on reducing this cost supports the inclusion of the therapies designed and provided at the Stroke Recovery Center to long-term care programs for stroke survivors throughout the country.

Falls

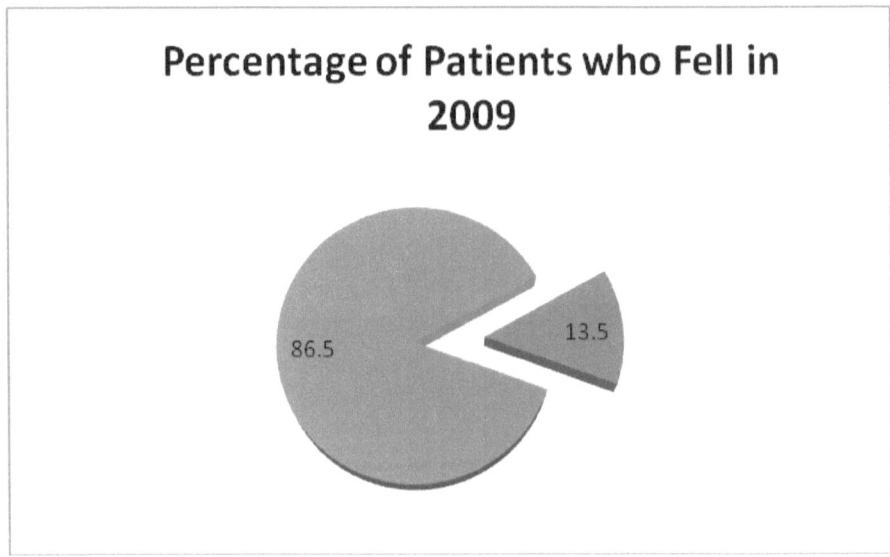

The overall numbers continue to decline to 13.5% of patients suffering falls in 2009 as compared to 20.4% and 30% in the prior years. This current number is well below the national norm for seniors, which is 30%. Considering the client base is elderly and handicapped, the numbers show significant progress in treatment. The data shows a higher propensity to fall in the first two years of attendance at the center. Taken with the data points in calculating ambulation variation and orthotic use, falls are correlated to the increased use of ambulation assistance and training. The benefit of continuing care is quantifiable in cost reduction due to the secure mobility of the patient.

The cost reductions to the health-care system as a whole from the reduction of falls in the frail and elderly are significant not only in the medical cost, the hospital cost, and the medication cost but also in elements like first-responder cost and lost productivity of caregivers needed for recovery. This statistic by itself supports the inclusion of the therapies of the center in a long-term care plan for stroke survivors throughout the country.

CONCLUSIONS

We have seen some significant shifts in data sets over the three years of this study that begin to point in directions that correlate some of the therapies to outcomes both expected and unexpected. Additionally, the study allows us to identify shortcomings of the center and determines what changes should be made going forward to better ensure the success of the patients in attaining and maintaining maximum feasible functionality.

The age of the patient base shows that we concentrate in the high-propensity age bracket of 60–79 years of age. It is in this age bracket that men and women are equal in the prevalence of stroke. Prior to that age, women are twice as likely to have strokes than men. That said, one might expect that the center has a higher level of participation from women, which holds true only in the first 2 years of attendance and then switches to a preponderance of men. Additionally, there is a limited group of 80+ attendees where the stoke risk is much higher. This suggests that there may need to be a different level of services available to the frail older patients as well as the female patients to bring the numbers more in line with the national stroke statistics.

The drug usage study indicates the wide variety of prescription drugs that are used. A number of patients are very heavy drug users due to comorbidities, such as HIV/AIDS. Additionally, there are a number of patients who are heavy users of dietary supplements. The average numbers are equal to the Kaiser study of senior prescription drug usage; however, individual drug usage and interactions may be putting the patients at risk.

Transportation is an area that continues the trend first noted in year 1 of the study. As the patients continue to participate at the center, they become less reliant on family to provide transportation and begin to rely on publicly available services or return to being able to transport themselves. Nonfamily-caregiver dependency stays constant. Of the long-term cost of stroke, a significant portion is due to lack of family productivity caused by the necessity for family caregivers. Long-term cost of stroke is estimated at $140,048 per survivor, only $13,019–$20,346 of which is expended in the first thirty days following the episode.

The major decreases in falls from the patient base need to be correlated with the increased use of orthotics and ambulatory aids that are evident as the patients stay in treatment with the exercise therapists. The concentration is on balance and strength building, both of which do require time to be effective. With a fall rate of only 13.5% in an elderly handicapped population, the effectiveness of treatment is supported. Initial studies indicated that there was less use of orthotics and ambulatory aids as the years off attendance increased; however, over time, the data indicates a more aggressive use of aids to help in mobility in conjunction with exercise. The results clearly support the cost effectiveness of using the aids to reduce falls and increase confident mobility. Falls are a major cost factor in elderly and frail populations, not only due to ER fees, but also resultant hospitalizations, nursing home days, home visits, and loss of productivity.

Emergency room (ER) visits are a major segment of cost to the healthcare system as a whole. While the patients who are in the first 2 years of attendance tend to be closer to their initial episodes and, therefore, have a higher likelihood of having been in the ER, as they remain at the center, the propensity to use the ER declines sharply until end-of-life issues intervene. The usage follows a bell-shaped curve with heavy use in the early and last years of attendance. The ability to influence the early use is limited as, in most cases, the patient is unknown. However, it might be possible to have a greater influence on the end-of-life choices that are made by the patients. Currently, this is not included in the educational program except on a one- to two-time-per-year educational session on advance directives.

The data has strongly supported the efforts of the Stroke Recovery Center but suggests that the center is only taking the first steps to assist their patients on their recovery. The data supports the creation of an environment in which healing can take place and where patients can gain some control over their lives, regaining some of the skills and independence they enjoyed prior to the stroke or TBI. The data further supports the value of exercise in increasing secure mobility that in turn adds to confidence and independence. However, on the other hand, the data also suggests that patient-focused care should be instituted to maximize value for each individual patient. Cost savings to the system should be allocated to support this case management and program development and need to be garnered from the sources that benefit. There are clear and undeniable data to support this notion, and it is the clear direction that the studies have revealed.

SAMPLE MENU

Mon	Tue	Wed	Thu	Fri
2 BBQ Pork Sandwich Coleslaw Dessert	3 Quiche Salad Roll Dessert	4 Chicken Ala King Rice & Veges Roll Dessert	5 **SRC CLIENT OUTING**	6 Pasta & M... Salad Garlic Br... Dessert
9 Tuna Salad Sandwich Fries Dessert	10 Turkey Tetrazzini Rice & Veges Dessert	11 Salisbury Steak Potato & Veges Roll Dessert	12 Chicken Waldorf Salad Roll Dessert	13 Baked Til... Rice & Ve... Roll Dessert
16 "Kicked Up" Mac & Cheese Tossed Salad Roll	17 Asian Chicken Salad Roll Dessert	18 Vege Lasagna Salad Roll Dessert	19 Burgers Fries Dessert	20 Beef Strog... Buttered ... Veges & ... Dessert
23 Stuffed Peppers Potato Roll Dessert	24 Lemon Chicken Cutlet Potato & Veges Roll Dessert	25 Fiesta Taco Salad Bowl Dessert	26 BBQ Ribs Corn on the Cobb Potato Salad Dessert	27 Crab Cak... Rice & Ve... Roll Dessert
30 **MEMORIAL DAY** **SRC CLOSED**	31 Greek Chicken Salad Roll Dessert			Menu Sub... without no...

SAMPLE ACTIVITIES CALENDAR

MONDAY	TUESDAY	WEDNESDAY	THURSDAY	FRIDAY
2	3	4	5	6
8:30 Social Hour	8:30 Social Hour	8:30 Social Hour	**OUTING**	8:30 Social Hour
9:30 Table Interactions	9:30 Table Interactions	9:30 Table Interactions	**Bird Rescue Sanctuary**	9:30 Table Interactions
10:30 Memory Bear Group	10:30 Word Power-Paul	10:00 Rap Session-Colleen		10:30 Word Power-Paul
11:30 Meditation & Relaxation	12:00 Wii Game Therapy	11:30 Music		11:45 Music-Conjunto
12:30 Lunch	12:30 Lunch	12:30 Lunch		12:30 Lunch
1:30 Wii Game Family Feud	1:30 Trivia	1:15 Bingo		1:15 Bingo
9	10	11	12	13
8:30 Social Hour	8:30 Social Hour	8:30 Social Hour	8:30 Social Hour	8:30 Social Hour
9:30 Table Interactions	9:30 Table Interactions	9:30 Table Interactions	9:30 Life Changes-Cedric King	9:30 Table Interactions
10:30 Photo of The Month Contest	10:30 Word Power-Paul	10:30 Rap Session-Colleen	10:30 Art Through Words Grp.	10:30 Word Power-Paul
11:30 Caren Doll's Dance Therapy	12:00 Wii Game Therapy	11:00 Animal Samaritans	11:30 Wii Game Therapy	11:45 Music
12:30 Lunch	12:30 Lunch	11:30 Music-Diva Denise	12:30 Lunch	12:30 Lunch
1:30 Trivia	1:30 Trivia	12:30 Lunch	1:30 Trivia	1:15 Bingo
		1:15 Bingo		

16
8:30 Social Hour
9:30 Table Interactions
10:30 Memory Bear Grp.
11:30 **Alzheimer's Assoc. Speaker**
12:30 Lunch
1:30 Wii Game Jeopardy

17
8:30 Social Hour
9:30 Table Interactions
10:30 Word Power-Paul
11:30 **Desert Samaritans Speaker**
12:30 Lunch
1:30 Trivia

18
8:30 Social Hour
9:30 Table Interactions
10:30 Rap Session-Colleen
11:30 **County of Riverside Speaker**
12:30 Lunch
1:15 Bingo

19
8:30 Social Hour
9:30 Table Interactions
11:30 **Eisenhower Smilow Heart Assoc.**
12:30 Lunch
1:30 Trivia

20
8:30 Social Hour
9:30 **Stroke Center Health Fair**
11:30 **Mayor Pougnet Presentation**
12:30 Lunch
1:15 Bingo

STROKE AWARENESS WEEK

23
8:30 Social Hour
9:30 Table Interactions
10:30 Memory Bear Grp.
11:30 Music-Al Apodaca
12:30 Lunch
1:30 Wii Game Family Feud

24
8:30 Social Hour
9:30 Table Interactions
10:30 Word Power-Paul
12:00 Wii Game Therapy
12:30 Lunch
1:30 Trivia

25
8:30 Social Hour
9:30 Table Interactions
10:30 Rap Session-Colleen
11:00 Animal Samaritans
11:45 Music-Mark G.
12:30 Lunch
1:15 Bingo
Pajama Party

26
8:30 Social Hour
9:30 Life Changes-Cedric King
10:30 Art Through Words Grp.
12:30 Lunch
1:30 Trivia

27
8:30 Social Hour
9:30 Table Interactions
10:30 Word Power-Paul
11:45 Music-Dixie Cats
12:30 Lunch
1:15 Bingo

30
MEMORIAL DAY
SRC CLOSED

31
8:30 Social Hour
9:30 Table Interactions
10:30 Word Power-Paul
12:00 Wii Game Therapy
12:30 Lunch
1:30 Trivia

Calendar events are subject to change without advanced warning.

WEBSITE

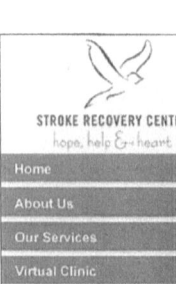

STATS REPORT

STROKE RECOVERY CENTER - DEPARTMENTS REPORT

FY 2010
OVERALL THERAPY PROGRAMS

CLIENTS SERVED (during last 12 months) 235 256 (Prior FY)

	JUL	AUG	SEP	OCT	NOV	DEC	JAN	FEB	MAR	APR	MAY	JUN	FYTD	Prior FYTD	Prior FY	
TOTAL CLIENTS SERVED	93	97	108	110	106	108	120	114	112				108	107	107	(Average)
TOTAL VISITS	660	721	792	822	804	783	886	798	917				7183	6902	9186	(Total)
DAYS OPEN PER MONTH	21	22	21	21	20	21	21	19	23				189	188	252	(Total)
AVERAGE DAILY VISITS	31	33	40	39	40	37	42	42	40				38	37	36	(Average)
PRIOR FY	33	35	36	36	36	35	40	40	39	36	38	33				

VISITS PER MONTH

	JUL	AUG	SEP	OCT	NOV	DEC	JAN	FEB	MAR	APR	MAY	JUN	FYTD	Prior FYTD	Prior FY	
1-2 VISITS	18	21	25	21	21	25	20	19	20				21	27	27	(Average)
3-5 VISITS	27	21	23	25	18	26	26	26	17				23	23	23	(Average)
6-10 VISITS	28	32	33	42	38	32	35	50	43				37	30	30	(Average)
11-15 VISITS	11	14	19	12	17	15	23	12	18				16	18	17	(Average)
16+ VISITS	9	9	8	12	12	10	10	7	14				10	10	10	(Average)
NEW CLIENTS	5	5	10	7	7	14	6	4	6				64	97	124	(Total)
WEBSITE VISITORS	1525	1596	1320	391	325	430	336	462					6385			(Total)
	(Total hits)			(Non-admin visitors)												

EXERCISE THERAPY

	JUL	AUG	SEP	OCT	NOV	DEC	JAN	FEB	MAR	APR	MAY	JUN	FYTD	Prior FYTD	Prior FY	
TOTAL CLIENTS	82	82	86	91	91	93	105	97	99				92	87	87	(Average)
% of Therapy Pgm. Clients	88%	85%	80%	83%	86%	86%	88%	85%	88%				85%	81%	81%	
TOTAL VISITS	490	534	580	628	606	555	630	607	632				585	561	563	(Average)
AVERAGE DAILY VISITS	23	25	29	31	30	28	32	34	29				29	28	28	(Average)
PRIOR FY	26	23	24	26	25	21	23	21	27	27	27	25				

SPEECH THERAPY

	JUL	AUG	SEP	OCT	NOV	DEC	JAN	FEB	MAR	APR	MAY	JUN	FYTD	Prior FYTD	Prior FY	
TOTAL CLIENTS	11	9	17	23	19	14	24	22	22				18	14	14	(Average)
% of Therapy Pgm. Clients	12%	9%	16%	21%	18%	13%	20%	19%	20%				17%	13%	13%	
TOTAL VISITS	32	32	40	74	61	61	104	101	95				67	46	46	(Average)
AVERAGE DAILY VISITS	2	2	2	4	3	3	5	6	4				3	2	2	
PRIOR FY	3	3	4	4	4	3	3	5	4	3	5	3				

MEAL PROGRAM

	JUL	AUG	SEP	OCT	NOV	DEC	JAN	FEB	MAR	APR	MAY	JUN	FYTD	Prior FYTD	Prior FY	
TOTAL CLIENT MEALS	296	331	363	357	364	317	375	306	366				3075	3368	4320	(Total)
CLIENTS SERVED	46	50	51	53	49	51	56	54	53				51	54	53	(Average)
% of Therapy Pgm. Clients	49%	52%	47%	48%	46%	47%	47%	47%	47%				48%	50%	49%	
TOTAL MEALS SERVED	698	736	693	761	733	660	742	678	777				6478	6941	9042	(Total)
AVERAGE DAILY MEALS	33	33	33	36	37	31	35	36	34				34	37	36	

VOLUNTEER PROGRAM												
HOURS												
Administration	173	140	145	123	112	117	132	102	122	1163	1135	1576	(Total)
Exercise Therapy	88	94	103	126	129	82	95	85	120	920	835	1130	(Total)
Fundraising													
Kitchen	721	706	386	571	541	519	560	623	740	5364	4735	6381	(Total)
Outreach													
Rec. Therapy	98	254	194	149	206	180	103	127	137	1446	1000	1364	(Total)
Speech Therapy	67	80	91	120	113	103	128	113	116	930	762	1086	(Total)
Thrift Shop	385	292	397	415	354	383	363	426	602	3615	3930	5000	(Total)
TOTAL HOURS	1530	1564	1314	1503	1453	1383	1381	1475	1836	13437	12397	16535	(Total)
VOLUNTEERS													
Administration	7	6	7	8	6	5	5	4	4	6	6	7	(Average)
Exercise Therapy	7	3	5	10	7	5	5	7	8	6	4	4	(Average)
Fundraising													
Kitchen	27	27	19	28	24	33	31	30	26	27	26	26	(Average)
Outreach													
Rec. Therapy	14	16	18	11	15	19	17	19	23	17	19	19	(Average)
Speech Therapy	4	4	5	5	6	5	6	6	5	5	4	5	(Average)
Thrift Shop	15	11	15	17	13	17	12	14	16	14	15	15	(Average)
TOTAL VOLUNTEERS	74	67	69	79	71	84	76	80	82	76	74	75	(Average)

CLIENT PROFILE

CLIENTS SERVED	93	97	108	110	106	108	120	114	112	189	%	256
INCOME LEVEL												
X-Low (less than $22,750 per year)	44	49	52	54	48	52	53	52	55	87	46%	114
Low ($22,750 - $36,400 per year)	19	18	20	22	23	20	22	26	23	41	22%	56
Moderate ($36,400 - $52,650 per year)	12	14	17	19	17	17	20	16	18	27	14%	38
High (over $52,650 per year)	18	16	19	15	18	19	25	20	16	34	18%	30
CITY OF RESIDENCE												
Banning/Beaumont/Cherry Valley	0	0	0	0	0	0	0	0		0	0%	3
Bermuda Dunes	0	0	0	0	0	0	1	1		1	1%	2
Cathedral City	23	26	26	26	24	24	22	23	23	32	17%	45
Coachella	0	1	1	1	0	0	0	2	1	2	1%	5
Desert Hot Springs	14	12	14	14	11	16	16	18	15	28	15%	35
Indian Wells	0	0	1	1	1	0	2	1	1	2	1%	1
Indio	4	4	4	6	5	7	8	5	6	9	5%	13
La Quinta	2	3	4	3	3	4	5	3	4	5	3%	7
Palm Desert	9	10	9	10	11	10	13	11	12	20	11%	30
Palm Springs	30	27	35	35	39	34	37	38	36	60	32%	75
Rancho Mirage	5	4	4	6	6	6	6	6	6	12	6%	12
San Jacinto/Hemet/Temecula/Winchester	2	2	1	2	1	1	1	1	1	2	1%	4
Thousand Palms	1	2	2	2	2	2	3	1	2	3	2%	5
Morongo/Joshua Tree/Yucca Valley/29 Palms	1	2	2	1	1	0	1	0	1	2	1%	8
Other	2	4	5	3	2	4	6	4	3	11	6%	11
GENDER												
Male	62	62	66	63	64	69	73	69		114	60%	158
Female	31	35	42	47	42	39	47	45		75	40%	98
ETHNICITY												
Anglo/White	70	71	79	82	82	82	95	89		143	76%	192
Hispanic	14	15	17	17	15	19	18	19		34	18%	40
Black/African American	6	7	8	7	5	4	5	3		8	4%	16
American Indian/Alaskan Native	0	0	0	0	0	0	0	0		0	0%	1
Asian/Pacific Islands	3	4	4	4	4	3	2	3		4	2%	7
AGE												
Under 35 years of age	2	2	3	4	3	2	0	1		4	2%	4
35 - 54 years of age	13	17	17	17	17	18	17	16		29	15%	39
55 - 74 years of age	45	46	56	55	54	53	63	59		84	44%	117
75 and Older	33	32	32	34	32	35	40	38		72	38%	96

BIBLIOGRAPHY

Agawin, Madelia. *Healing Fields.* Xlibris Corporation, 2008.

Bauby, Jean-Dominique. *The Diving Bell and the Butterfly.* New York: Alfred A. Knopf, 1997.

Braley, Doris W. *Stroke: The Road Back.* Portland: Harbor House West, 1994.

Doidge, Norman. *The Brain that Changes Itself.* New York: the Penguin Group, 2007.

Garrison, Julia Fox. *Don't Leave Me This Way.* New York: Harper, 2007.

Shapiro, Alison Bonds. *Healing into Possibility.* Tiberon, CA: HJ Kramer, 2009.

Stroke Brain-Assault. Nevada City, CA: Blue Dolphin Publishing, 2002.

Taylor, Jill Bolte. *My Stroke of Insight.* New York: the Penguin Group, 2006.

Timothy, Megan. *Let Me Die Laughing!.* Idyllwild, CA: Crone House Publishing, 2006.

Internet References

"Traumatic Brain Injury," Wikipedia.org

"Heart Disease and Stroke Statistics—2010 Update," American Heart Association.org

Susan Jeffrey, "Total US Stroke Costs for 2005–2050 Projected to Reach $2.2 Trillion," *Medscape Medical* "News," medscape.com

"Stroke Statistics," the University Hospital, umdnj.edu

"Caregiver Statistics," nfcacares.org, 2011

Post Stroke Rehabilitation Fact Sheet, *National Institute of Neurological Disorders and Stroke*, NIH Publication No. 08-4846

"What is Post Stroke Depression?," wiseGEEK.com

TBI Resource Guide, *Center for Neuro Skills*, neuroskills.com

"Stroke Care Giving," *Journal of Gerontological Nursing*, April 2006

Eden Alternative.org

"Tai Chi and Stroke Recovery," wingsunkungfuwear.com

"Curry Spice Could Aid in Stroke Recovery," ksat.com

"Magnetic Stimulation May Speed Stroke Rehab," WebMD.com

"Stress Management Center," WebMD.com

"Acupuncture Not Effective in Stroke Recovery," eurekalert.org

Stroke Rehab Getting Patients Back on Their Feet: Intensive Home Therapy As Good As 'High Tech,'" medicalnewstoday.com

"Designing Safety-net Clinics for Innovative Care Delivery Models," prepared by the Center for Health Design for California Healthcare Foundation, March 2011

INDEX

A

accountable care organizations 88, 90
activities of daily living x, 3, 10, 17, 18, 45, 72
acupuncture 49, 59, 72, 174
acute rehabilitation 16, 22, 98
    caregivers and 23
    occupational and recreational therapists and 18
    physical therapists and 17
    physicians and 16
    rehabilitation nurses and 17
    speech-language therapists and 19
    vocational therapists and 20
advocacy 64, 70, 79, 81, 83–85, 91
Affordable Care Act 79
Agawin, Madelina 50
    Healing Fields, The 50
AHA (American Heart Association) 30, 31, 83, 173
Americans with Disabilities Act of 1990 20
aphasia 4, 12, 19, 54
apraxia 13, 18
ataxia 11

B

Bauby, Jean-Dominique 6, 9, 19, 28, 33, 97, 98, 173
    Diving Bell and the Butterfly, The 6, 97, 98, 173

C

caregiving 27, 29, 32, 34–38
clinical depression 13

D

Diving Bell and the Butterfly, The (Bauby) 6, 97, 98, 173
Doidge, Norman 46, 99, 173
Don't Leave Me This Way (Garrison) 10, 97–99, 173
Duncan, Pamela W. 42

E

Eden Alternative 47, 174
exercises, types of 10
exercise therapy 39, 42, 58, 59, 110, 121, 154

G

Garrison, Julia Fox 10, 21, 29, 30, 34, 49, 97–99, 173
    Don't Leave Me This Way 10, 97–99, 173

H

Healing Fields, The (Agawin) 50
Healing into Possibility (Shapiro) 28, 97–99, 173
Hirshleifer, Irving 53
hydrotherapy 18

J

JCAHO (Joint Commission on Accreditation of Healthcare Organizations) 79
Journal of Gerontological Nursing 35, 174

K

Kahn-Feurer, Lois H. xi, 38

L

learned nonuse 17
locked-in syndrome 6, 7, 19, 33

M

Meade, Margaret xi
medical homes 87, 88
ministroke 4. *See* TIA (transient ischemic attack)
MOTOmed 59
My Stroke of Insight (Taylor) 7, 97–99, 173

N

National Stroke Association 30, 47, 49, 111

O

OHIP (Organizational Health Initiative Project) 103, 103–105, 109, 129–131, 135, 147–149, 153

P

PACE (Project for All-inclusive Care for the Elderly) 88, 89
PCS (postconcussion syndrome) 8
poststroke depression 13, 23, 24, 111
post-traumatic stress disorder 25
PTA (post-traumatic amnesia) 8

S

safety-net clinics 90, 174
Shapiro, Alison Bonds 28, 29, 33, 97–99, 173
    Healing into Possibility 28, 97–99, 173

socialization 34, 37, 62, 63, 65, 66
stroke ix, x, xi, 1, 3, 3–14, 16–40, 42–51, 53–58, 61, 62, 64, 65, 67, 70–75, 77–79, 83–91, 95, 97–99, 103–109, 111, 112, 114–118, 120, 122, 124–129, 131, 134–139, 144–147, 149, 151–155, 157–159, 163–166, 169, 173, 174
    costs of 83
    experience during 6
    problems of 71
        emotional disturbances 11, 13
        motor control 11
        sensory disturbances 10, 11
        thinking and memory 11, 13
        using or understanding language 11–12
    reaction of people with 9
    sources of help for 26
        community and organizations 29
        families and friends 27
    statistics of 3
    types of 3, 117
        hemorrhagic 3, 5, 6, 26, 117
        ischemic 3, 4, 26, 117
    warning signs of 5
Stroke Recovery Center ix, x, xi, 4, 5, 8, 16, 27, 29–32, 34, 37–40, 44–51, 53–58, 62, 70–75, 77, 78, 79, 84, 85, 87, 89–91, 103, 105–109, 111, 114, 116–118, 120, 124–127, 129, 131, 135, 136, 144, 146, 147, 149, 151, 153, 154, 163, 166
    advocacy and 85–87
    alternative therapies of 49–50
    barriers to development in 77–79
    constraints of 72
    development of 73–74
    history of 53–54
    leadership in 75–76
    needs of 71
    philosophy of 55–57
    programs and services provided in 71, 72

exercise therapy 58–60
food program 68–69
recreational therapy 62–68
speech and language therapy 61–62
research by 39–44

T

Taylor, Jill Bolte 7, 35, 97–99, 173
My Stroke of Insight 7, 97–99, 173
TBI (traumatic brain injury) ix, xi, 1, 3–6, 4, 8, 9, 13–16, 20–22, 24, 25, 27, 29–31, 35, 37–39, 44, 46–48, 56–58, 64, 65, 70–72, 74, 83–88, 91, 97, 137, 138, 149, 152, 157, 166, 173, 174

causes of 4
common diagnoses of 4
levels of 9, 35
problems of 13–16
symptoms of 8
TENS (transcutaneous electrical nerve stimulation) 18
thalamic pain syndrome 12
TIA (transient ischemic attack) 4
Timothy, Megan 22, 173

V

virtual clinic 31, 47, 54, 91

www.ingramcontent.com/pod-product-compliance
Lightning Source LLC
Chambersburg PA
CBHW032009170526
45157CB00002B/612